MAN

vs.

HAIR

Running Press
Hachette Book Group
1290 Avenue of the Americas, New York, NY 10104
www.runningpress.com
@Running_Press

Printed in China

First Edition: October 2017

Published by Running Press, an imprint of Perseus Books, LLC, a subsidiary of Hachette Book Group, Inc.

The Hachette Speakers Bureau provides a wide range of authors for speaking events. To find out more, go to www. hachettespeakersbureau.com or call (866) 376-6591.

The publisher is not responsible for websites (or their content) that are not owned by the publisher.

Library of Congress Control Number: 2017943619

ISBNs: 978-0-7624-6249-0 (hardcover),
978-0-7624-6250-6 (ebook)
CC062017
10 9 8 7 6 5 4 3 2 1

Publisher: Mark Searle
Editorial Director: Isheeta Mustafi
Commissioning Editor: Alison Morris
Editor: Angela Koo
Junior Editor: Abbie Sharman
Art Director: Michelle Rowlandson
Cover Design: Michelle Rowlandson
Book layout: Lucy Smith and Ian Miller
Illustrations: Sarah Skeate
Photography: Emma Gutteridge and Neal Grundy

Cover Image Credit:
Verity Jane Smith, Getty Images

MAN

vs.

HAIR

60

*Tutorials
for Handsome
Hair & Stubble*

KIERON WEBB

Running Press
PHILADELPHIA

CONTENTS

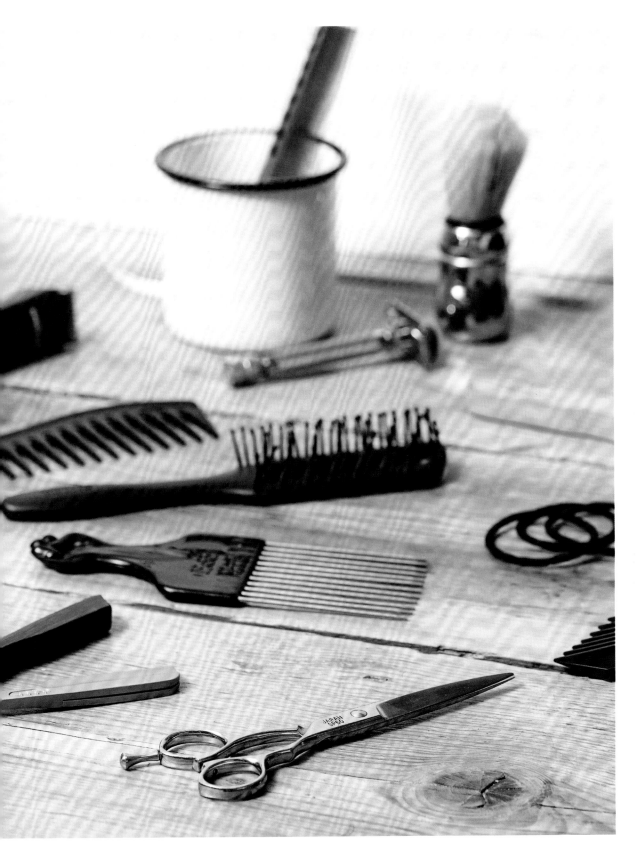

VISUAL DIRECTORY

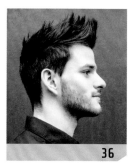 36

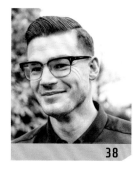 38

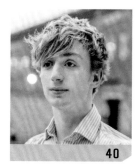 40

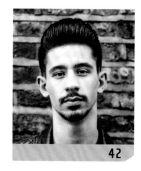 42

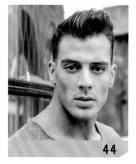 44

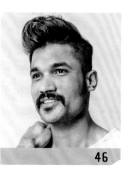 46

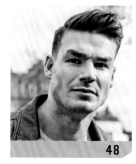 48

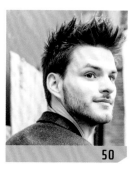 50

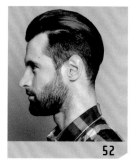 52

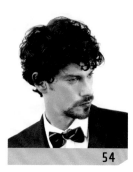 54

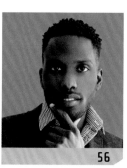 56

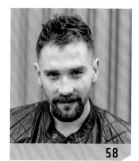 58

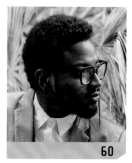 60

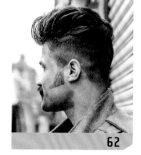 62

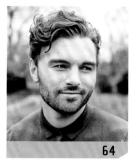 64

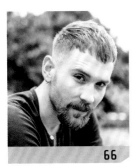 66

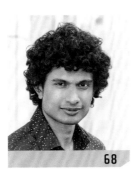 68

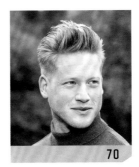 70

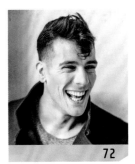 72

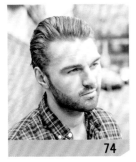 74

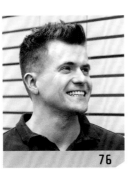 76

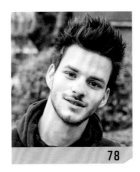 78

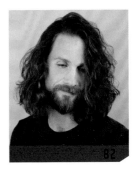 82

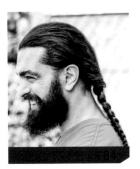 84

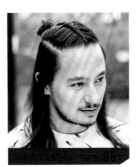 86

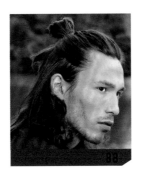 88

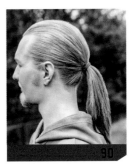 90

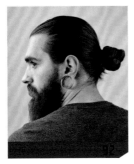 92

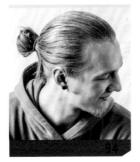 94

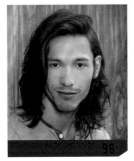 96

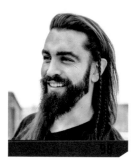

98

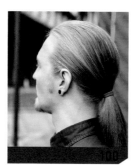

100

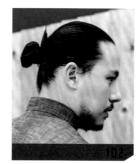

102

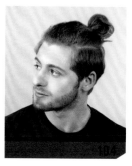

104

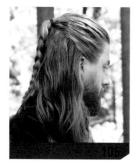

106

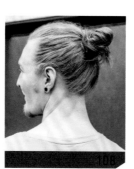

108

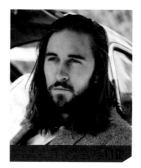

110

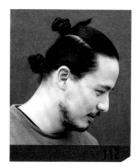

112

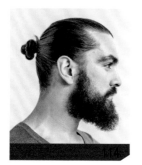

114

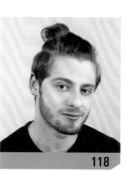

118

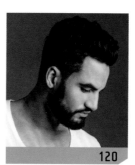

120

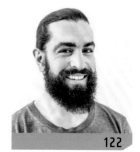

122

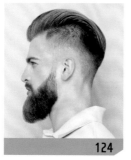

124

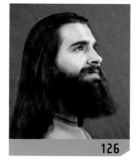

126

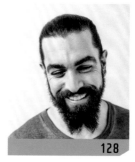

128

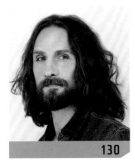 130

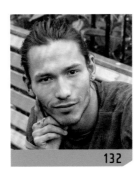 132

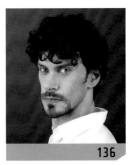 134

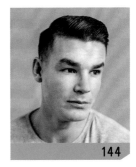 136

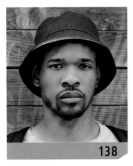 138

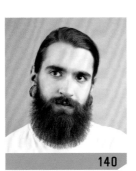 140

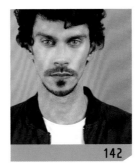 142

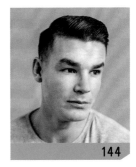 144

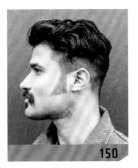 150

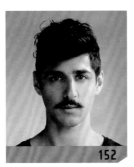 152

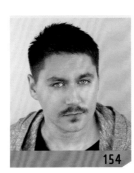 154

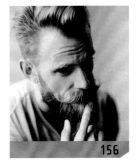 156

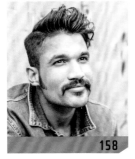 158

 160

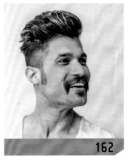 162

INTRODUCTION

I cut and style a lot of hair, and one of the things I notice a lot is that while guys will often have a very clear idea of the style they want, they are usually really surprised to discover the tools and products it will take to achieve it. There is often a lot more to a style than you think. But the good news is that this can all be learned.

It all comes down to practice, and not being afraid to have a go. I may travel the world, styling celebrity hair, but it took me 15 years of hard work to get where I am now, so if anyone knows the value of experience, it's me! But I have also tried to keep things simple because I wanted the styles in this book to be achievable. This is why you will find very few looks classified as "difficult"—I know plenty of people will see that word and be put off having a go (although I have included one or two in there for those of you who like a challenge). I have also broken down each style into no more than five stages so that you can follow through step by step, and at your own pace.

You will see a variety of different models throughout this book, too, so you're sure to spot someone who has similar hair to you. Some of these guys are friends of mine—professional models that I've worked with for years—but you definitely don't need to be in the industry to achieve similar looks with your own hair. In fact, I would stress that the most important thing is to respect your own look and personal style.

With trial and error, you'll get very familiar with your own hair. You can choose to wear it longer or shorter, but the one thing that you won't be able to change is its natural texture. You need to respect what you can achieve, and then work with that. Make sure, too, that you take into account the shape of your face, and how your hairstyle will work with that. Some styles will work on all hair types, too, so don't be afraid to experiment and try something different, even if the model's hair isn't the same as yours. It's your choice.

Above all, make the most of your strengths, and express who you are, not someone else. And have fun!

Kieron Hebb

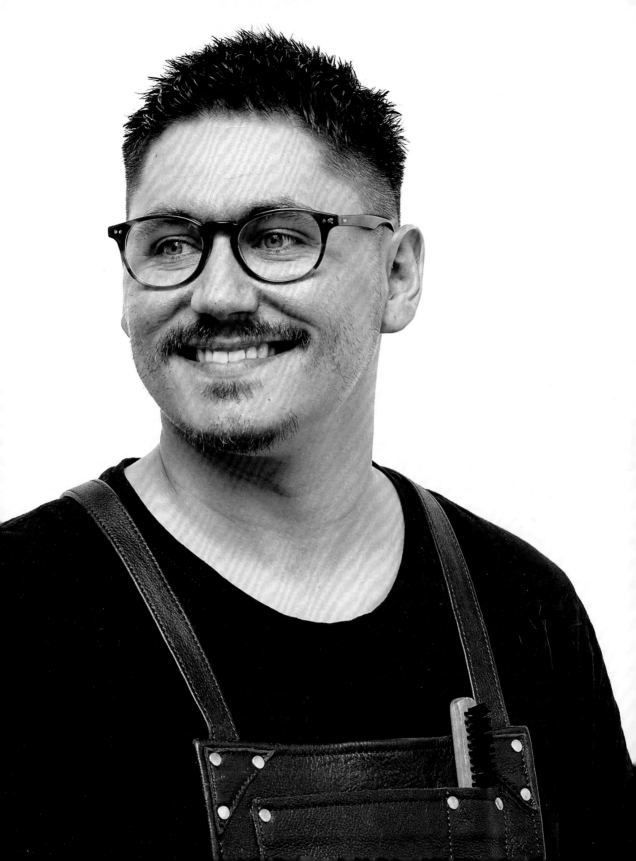

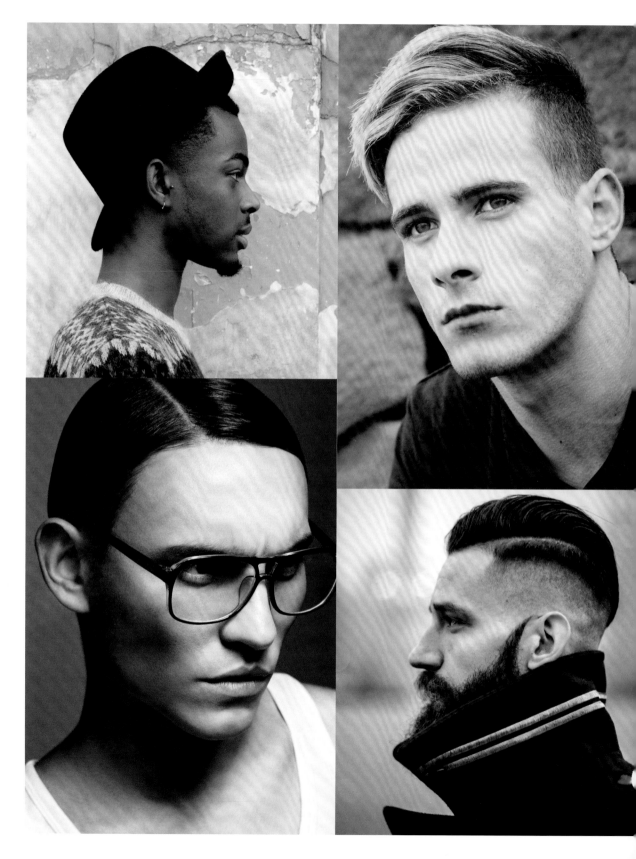

CHAPTER 1

SHORTER CUTS

Men will always want short hair—it's a classic "masculine" look that will never go out of style. However, there are many options to choose from, depending on your natural hair texture and your lifestyle. And, as you'll discover in this book, having a short cut won't mean that you can't express yourself in lots of different ways!

A short cut can range from the shortest of all—a buzz cut that takes it right back to a few millimeters—through to styles like crew cuts, and then on to fades and undercuts (see pages 62 and 76), where the hair on top can be as long as you like. And, within these categories, the length of the hair and the style can vary hugely.

RESPECT WHAT YOU'VE GOT
The main consideration for any successful cut will be your hair texture. You should always work with what you've got, not against it. Although tools and products can achieve a lot, they can't work miracles.

If you have straight hair, for example, you may decide to go for a classic, short cut that is easy to maintain. If you have curly hair, then why not leave a bit of length on top so that you can create textured looks that take advantage of your hair's natural volume? When it comes to Afro hair, there are dozens of different lengths to choose from, right down to a tight Afro, depending on what works with your face shape.

STYLING OPTIONS
Always take your lifestyle into account when choosing a style. If you work outdoors, for example, and don't have much time to spend on your hair, there's no point in going for a complicated cut that needs lots of styling. But having one cut definitely doesn't restrict you to just one style.

For example, take a look at the two different looks I created on my friend Tommy—the Textured Crop (page 58) and the Sleek Crop (page 66). These demonstrate just how much can be achieved with styling, even on very short hair. You can wear it as a neat forward crop during the day, then add a bit of product to transform it into the textured look for an evening out. Short hair like this also allows you to make a strong statement with your facial hair.

Above all, don't be afraid to experiment. Try a new cut, then play around with products to see what variations you can achieve. Look through this book, pick out something you like, and try it at least once. It's only through trial and error that you will learn what suits you best.

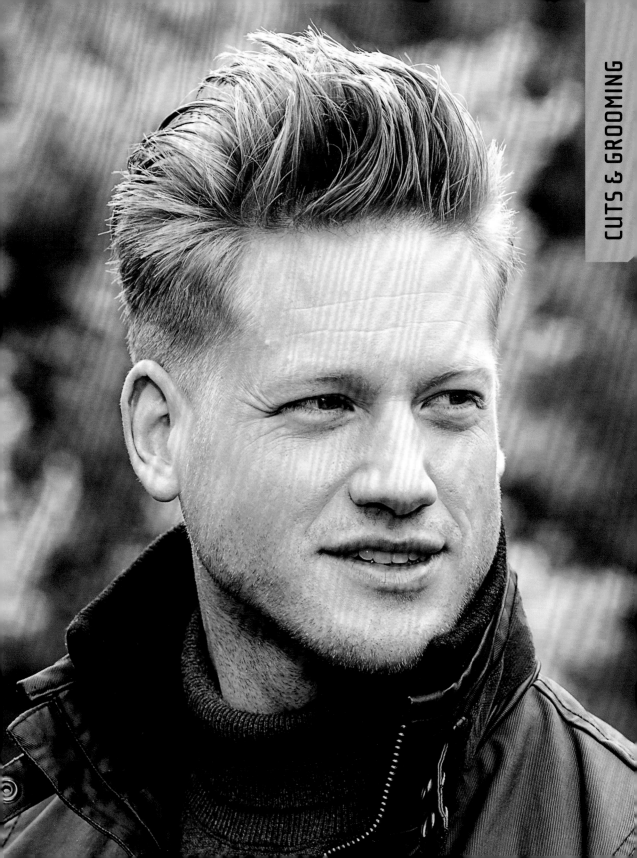

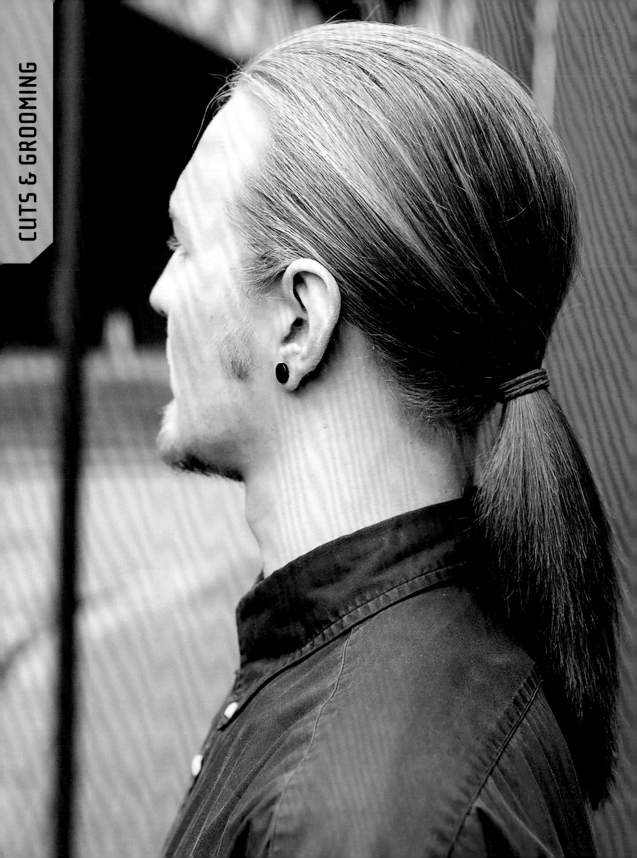

LONGER CUTS

Long hair comes in all shapes and sizes, from a mop top, as first worn by the Beatles, all the way through to hair that reaches way beyond the shoulders. And the look can range from tailored to messy. For the purposes of this book, I have classified longer styles as those where the hair is at least chin length—long enough to create looks such as ponytails, braids, and buns.

HAIR MAINTENANCE

Longer cuts obviously require a bit more maintenance than a simple wash-and-go cut, simply because there is more hair to take care of! If you are wanting to create super-clean, sharp looks, then you'll need to make sure that your hair is in good condition, with no split ends to spoil the effect of a slick style. Choose a good shampoo and conditioner, especially if your hair is coarse or prone to dryness, and be sure to get your hair trimmed regularly.

It is also worth asking your barber or stylist for advice on how to create a look that best frames your face. Long hair doesn't have to be all one length.

STYLING OPTIONS

If you are prepared to take on the maintenance of long hair, then the payoff will be maximum versatility when it comes to styling. Once you've read this book and mastered the techniques I will show you, you will be able to braid your hair, tie it back, and coil it up—or all of the above, and in any combination.

Wear your hair down and messy, or slick it back and tie it in a tight pony paired with a suit for a groomed, formal appearance. You don't need short hair to look sharp and classic! And there are plenty of options for adding extra interest with no extra effort—see, for example, the "samurai" styles on pages 94 and 102 for just two quick ideas.

Even hair that reaches only to the middle of your face will be long enough to attempt something interesting. For example, one of my best-known clients, Zayn Malik, got a lot of attention for a topknot that I created for him one year. At the time, he had an undercut (see page 18), and the hair on top reached only to his ears. It was the contrast between the shaved area at the lower part of his head, with the tight, sleek topknot above it that made this "long" style so striking.

FADES AND UNDERCUTS

These are styles where the hair is longer on top and shorter below, although they can be created with all sorts of variations in actual length. They are incredibly popular right now because they are a very effective way of adding visual interest for very little maintenance.

Although fades and undercuts often overlap, there is a difference between these two terms, which is worth knowing before you visit your barber.

UNDERCUT VERSUS FADE

An undercut is any haircut that is longer on top and shorter below. A "disconnected" undercut is where there is a strict contrast between the two—with hair much longer on top, and the sides consistently much shorter. A fade describes any sort of graduation, so when this appears on an undercut it means that the hair on the sides gradually "fades" or tapers as it progresses down toward the ears and neck. There is a smooth transition in length.

PLACEMENT

The first thing that you need to decide on is the overall shape. With a high fade, for example, the short sides come right up to your temples. This will create a strong look, especially if you have some length or texture in the hair on top. A mid-fade starts around halfway up, so this is a slightly less extreme look. A low fade starts lower down.

LENGTH VARIATIONS

The first thing to decide is how close to the head you want your sides to be—anything from around 13 mm (using a number 4 guard) right down to shaved!—and what degree of graduation you prefer. There are no rules, and you can always play around with variations every time you get it trimmed.

You also have lots of options when it comes to the hair on top. You might want to keep this short and messy, or you may prefer to keep a bit of length in it so that you can create slicked-back styles, perhaps with a side part, or maybe long bangs. Try to take your hair texture into account, though, because although the sides will be fairly maintenance-free, this is the part of the haircut that will need to be styled.

Take a look through this book and you'll spot a few looks for inspiration, or go online and see what other variations are possible.

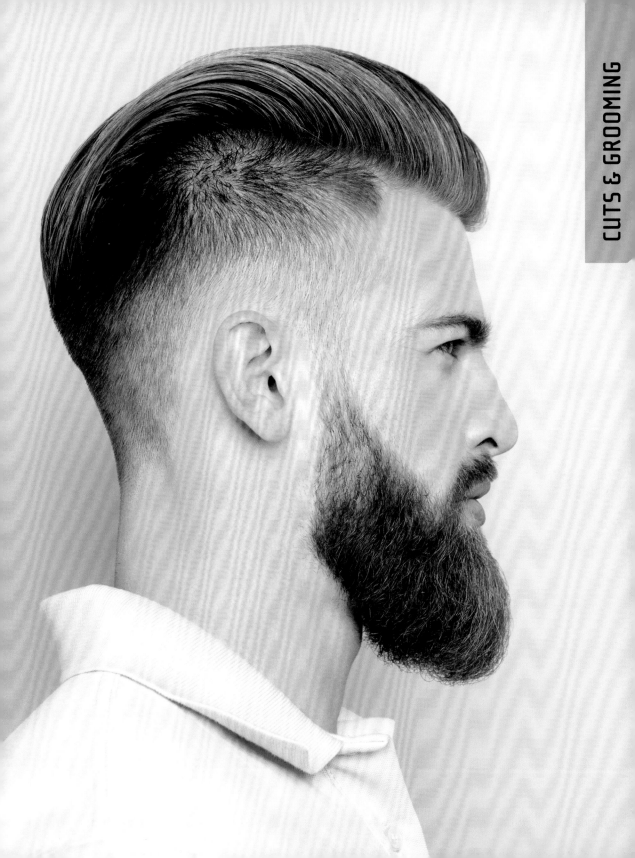

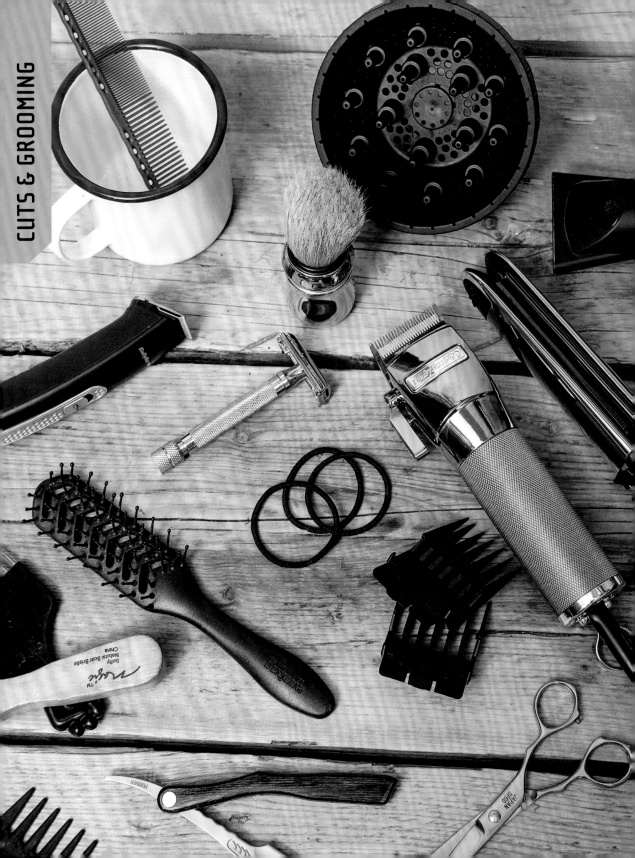

STYLING TOOLS

I can't count how many times a guy has come to me with a photo of a style they'd like, but when I've told them what they'll need to use to achieve it they've been shocked—they're usually expecting to be able to add a little product and go!

For this reason, I've kept it simple for the styles in this book. I know most of you will already have a comb, and probably a beard trimmer. And I daresay you'll have access to a hair dryer, too, even if it's something that you've done your best to avoid up til now! Here is a roundup of some of the basics...

WIDE-TOOTH AND SMALL-TOOTH COMB

A wide-tooth comb will glide easily through hair. It's perfect, too, for combing wet hair. A small-tooth comb is good for creating neat parts.

BRUSHES

There are lots of different brushes available, depending on the task. A round brush, for example, is great for creating a gentle curl in your hair while blow-drying; a plastic vent brush has wide-spaced bristles that allow for air flow when blow-drying; and a nylon/boar-bristle brush has amazing grip, is soft on the hair, and produces really smooth results when creating a ponytail.

AFRO PICK

The long, thin teeth on a pick are great for reaching right through thick layers of hair.

FLAT IRON OR HAIR STRAIGHTENER

A flat iron straightens and smooths out hair by clamping it between two metal plates. This process can also add texture to the hair, as you will see in some of the styles in this book.

HAIR DRYER

Most guys hate the idea of using a hair dryer, but this is one of the most useful tools of all, so learn to take advantage of it. The regular nozzle on your dryer will give a fuller, more directional blast of air. You can use this in combination with a brush to blow down the hair shaft, making the hair cuticle lie flat so that you get a smooth finish. Doing the opposite will ruffle the hair cuticle, creating a more voluminous effect. A diffuser attachment allows heat to come through, but not too much airflow, which is why it's good for curly hair, or when you want to avoid frizz.

BEARD TRIMMER

All beard trimmers come with a variety of guards (usually around eight) that you can swap to achieve your desired length. Make sure that you keep your blade oiled. All you need is three small dots of oil along the blade to maintain smooth movement between the moving metal parts.

RAZORS

A safety razor is so named because the blade is covered slightly—there is a buffer between the blade and your skin. A cut-throat razor is an open blade, so it can be easier to cut yourself, but as long as you are careful, this type of blade will give you the perfect close shave.

STYLING PRODUCTS

You may be surprised to discover what you'll need in terms of products to achieve most styles. Hair doesn't just magically do what you want it to! But you'll also be surprised at how quickly you can get to know the habits of your own hair and what works best for you.

A professional will have access to a huge selection of products, but for this book I've tried to keep it simple, so that you won't need to make a major investment to get started. What I've listed below are the products that I found myself reaching for most when creating the styles in this book, although I do mention other things along the way that aren't listed here—and, of course, you may also already have your own trusted favorites.

When it comes to quantity, this really depends on the length of your hair, and how thick it is, but gauging this for yourself will soon become second nature.

HAIRSPRAY

I am on a one-man mission when it comes to hairspray. Most men think hairspray is for women: this couldn't be more wrong. The sooner you embrace this styling product, the easier your life will be. Sprays range from soft to firm hold, and flexible hairspray is good when you need to be able to comb through the hair and layer on more spray as you go. Hold the can around 8 inches (20 cm) from your head and spray evenly. Go lightly, too—you can always add more.

POMADE

This is a great all-rounder, combining hold with a high-shine finish. Water-based pomades are lighter, whereas oil-based options are creamier and heavier. (The black product in the pot opposite is an example of a pomade—it's the exact one I used in this book.)

BEESWAX AND MATTE WAX

Beeswax-based products lock in moisture and give the hair plenty of shine. A little goes a long way. A matte wax will give a pliable but drier finish.

FIBER PASTE

This sticky paste is used to add texture, so is perfect for messy styles. Warming up the paste between your fingers will make it easy to work with; it will then cool and thicken on your hair, so you must apply it evenly.

SALT SPRAY

As the name suggests, this will give you a textured, tousled look, like you've just got back from the beach. It's very easy to apply, too.

CURL CREAM

This is a very useful product—it will define natural curls and prevent frizz.

AFTERSHAVE BALM

This is crucial step after shaving, to cool down the skin, reduce any irritation, and restore moisture. Look for a formulation to suit your skin type.

BEARD BALM / OIL

Both of these grooming products will soften and moisturize your beard—it depends on your preferred texture. A balm is a dense, creamy product that will also hold any stray hairs in place. Beard oil is lighter and more quickly absorbed. It will moisturize both your beard and your skin, so is great for shorter beards.

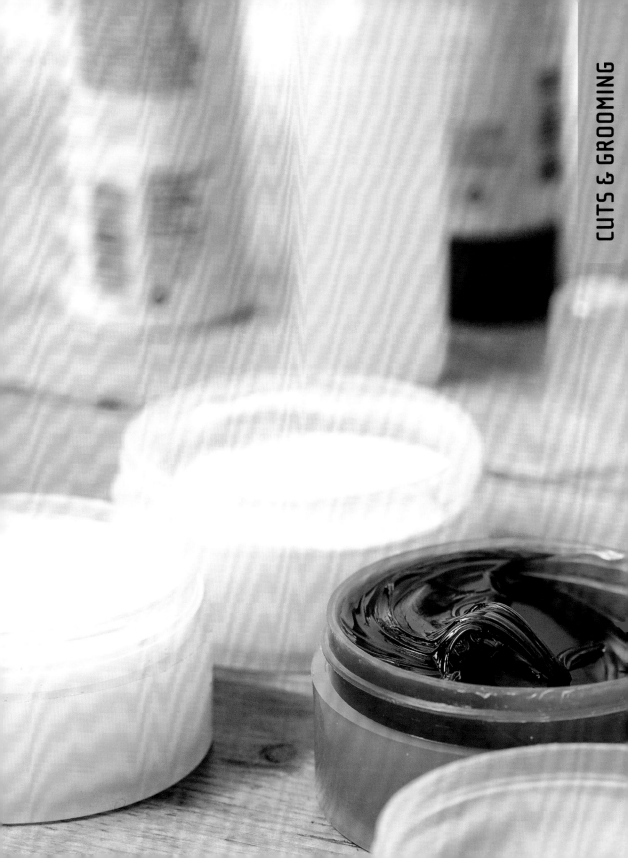

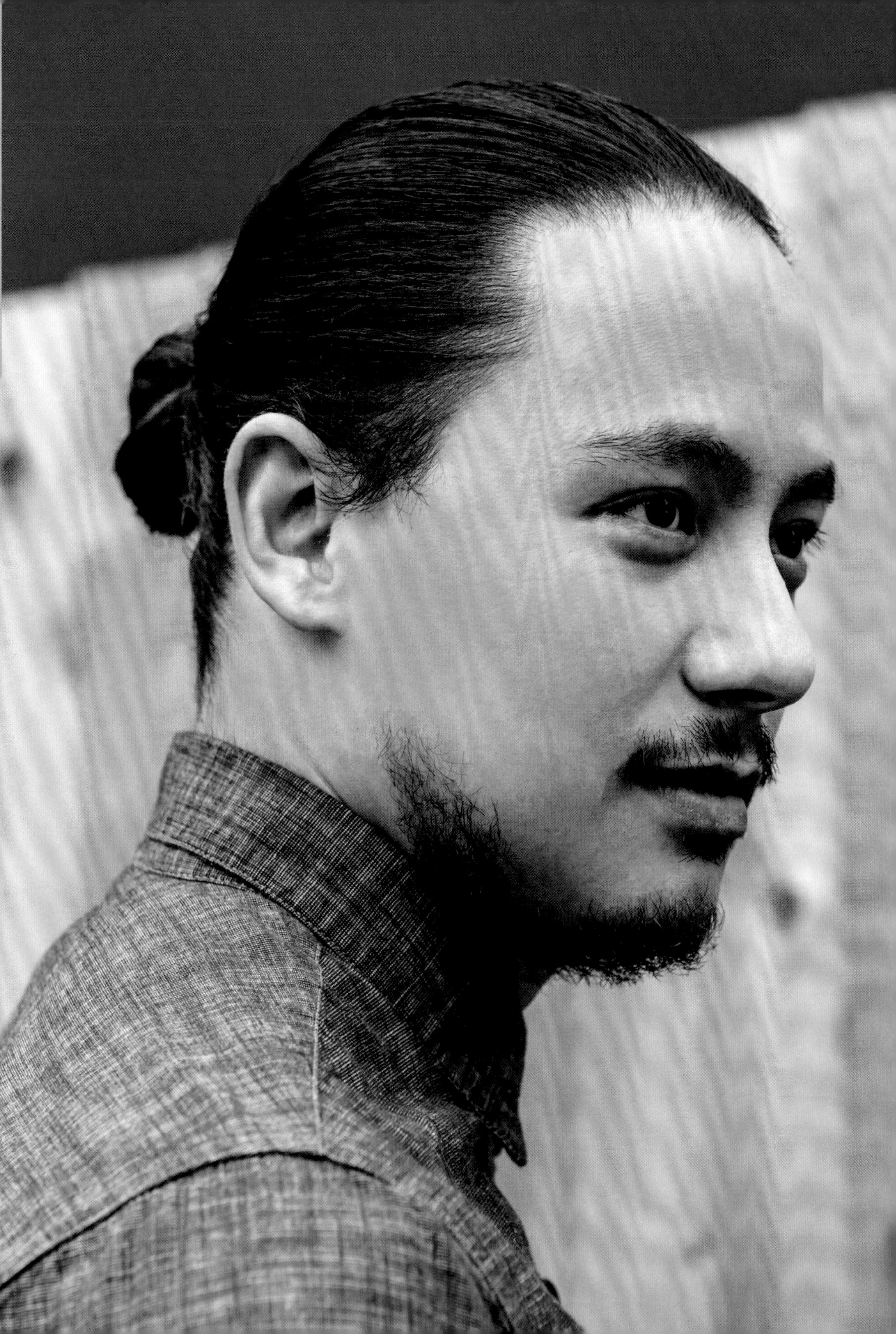

DOS AND DON'TS

I'm really passionate about education. When it comes to hair, getting the results you want is all about knowledge—knowing what tools and products are available and how to use them, as well as how to work effectively with the strengths and weaknesses of your own hair.

When I work with a lad who's looking for something new, I always make sure they go away with a clear understanding of the techniques I've used to create the look. This puts the power in their hands—they can then go away and recreate that same look by themselves at home. And that's why, with every style in this book, I've included practical tips for how to achieve the best results possible. But before you dive in, it's worth discussing a few basic dos and don'ts...

DO:
Get to know your hair dryer

I cannot stress this one enough, and it's something that you'll hear me repeat many times throughout the book. But I make no apologies for that! A hair dryer is one of the most important tools that you'll use. If you take the time to practice the techniques I describe, your hair dryer will end up doing a lot of the heavy lifting for you. It's always a matter of using your dryer in tandem with the correct brush, and working toward the desired shape right from the start, rather than trying to create it once your hair's already dry. And take note whenever I recommend using the diffuser attachment—this is for styles where you will need to use the heat of the dryer to set your hair in one position rather than blowing it all over the place.

DON'T:
Don't cut your own bangs...

...unless you really know what you're doing. You only need to look on YouTube to see why I warn against doing this! Cutting your bangs is not just a matter of cutting in a straight line; you need to know how to create a natural-looking line that follows the contours of your face. Beginners often pull their bangs down firmly to cut them, and are then surprised to discover that once they let go of the hair and it bounces back into place, the result is much shorter than intended.

DO:
Embrace hairspray

I'll put it simply. If you attempt even a simple style that requires hairspray but you try to dispense with the spray, then that style will go from "easy" to "difficult." You have been warned.

DON'T:
Randomly apply products to wet hair

Some products need to be applied to dry rather than wet hair. I make it clear in this book which product to use and at which stage of the process. Follow my instructions carefully to begin with and you'll soon have a good knowledge of which formulations work well with wet hair, and those that need to be applied after blow-drying.

DO:
Experiment

Don't feel that because the model shown for a particular style in this book doesn't have the same hair type as you, or that because your hair type isn't mentioned in the recommendations that I've given, that you can't try it anyway. It all comes down to trial and error—you need to explore new styles in order to discover new favorites. It's your hair: you're in control.

DOS AND DON'TS

DON'T:
Overload with product

Start with less rather than more. You can add but it isn't as easy to take away. Some products go a long way, so you only need the smallest drop. If you put too much oil through your hair, for example, you won't have shiny hair—you will have an oily mess.

DO:
Respect your hair type

Although it's worth exploring new looks, sometimes you'll have to accept that your hair just isn't suitable for a particular style. If you have tight curls, then no amount of product or styling will really achieve a smooth, flat-to-the head slickback, while dead-straight hair will never achieve the same volume and texture as curly hair.

DON'T:
Be afraid to tell your barber that you're unhappy with your haircut!

You need to be honest with them, and give them the chance to rectify it. And life is too short to live with a style that you're not happy with.

DO:
Practice, practice, and practice some more

If you don't get the right results the first time, keep trying. It takes a bit of repetition to get things looking perfect, especially when there's a new technique to master, like a braid. And if you've got an important event coming up and you want to try something new, take the stress out of the situation and make sure that you've tried it out beforehand.

DON'T:
Try to taper your own neckline

Get a professional to do it instead. And make sure that your barber doesn't give you a square neckline, either. It should taper, following the natural hairline along the neck.

DO:
Your research

Take advantage of all of the information available online and get to know the names of the various styles out there. When you come across a style that you like the look of in this book, then key it in and do a search for celebs wearing variations of the same thing. It will give you inspiration, and knowing the right terminology will help you communicate better with your barber or stylist, too.

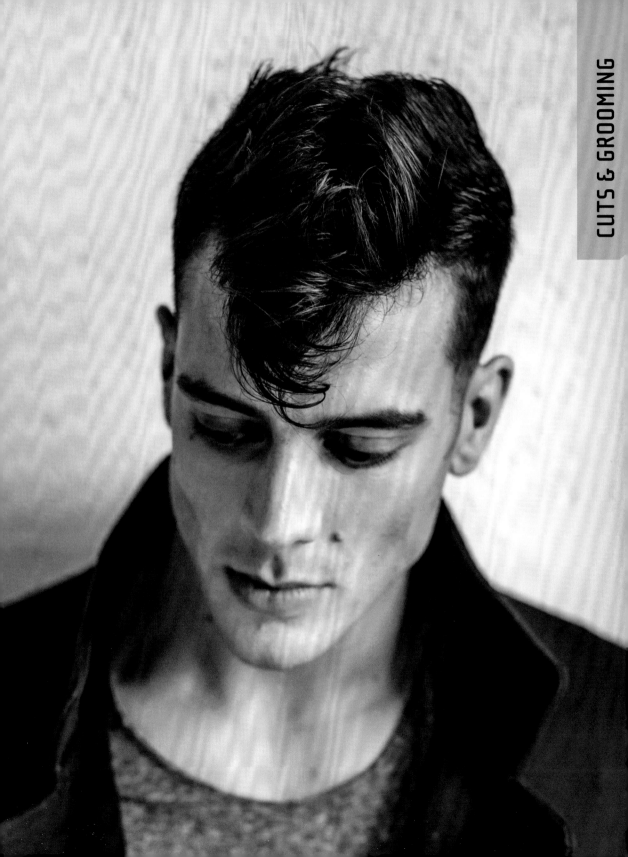

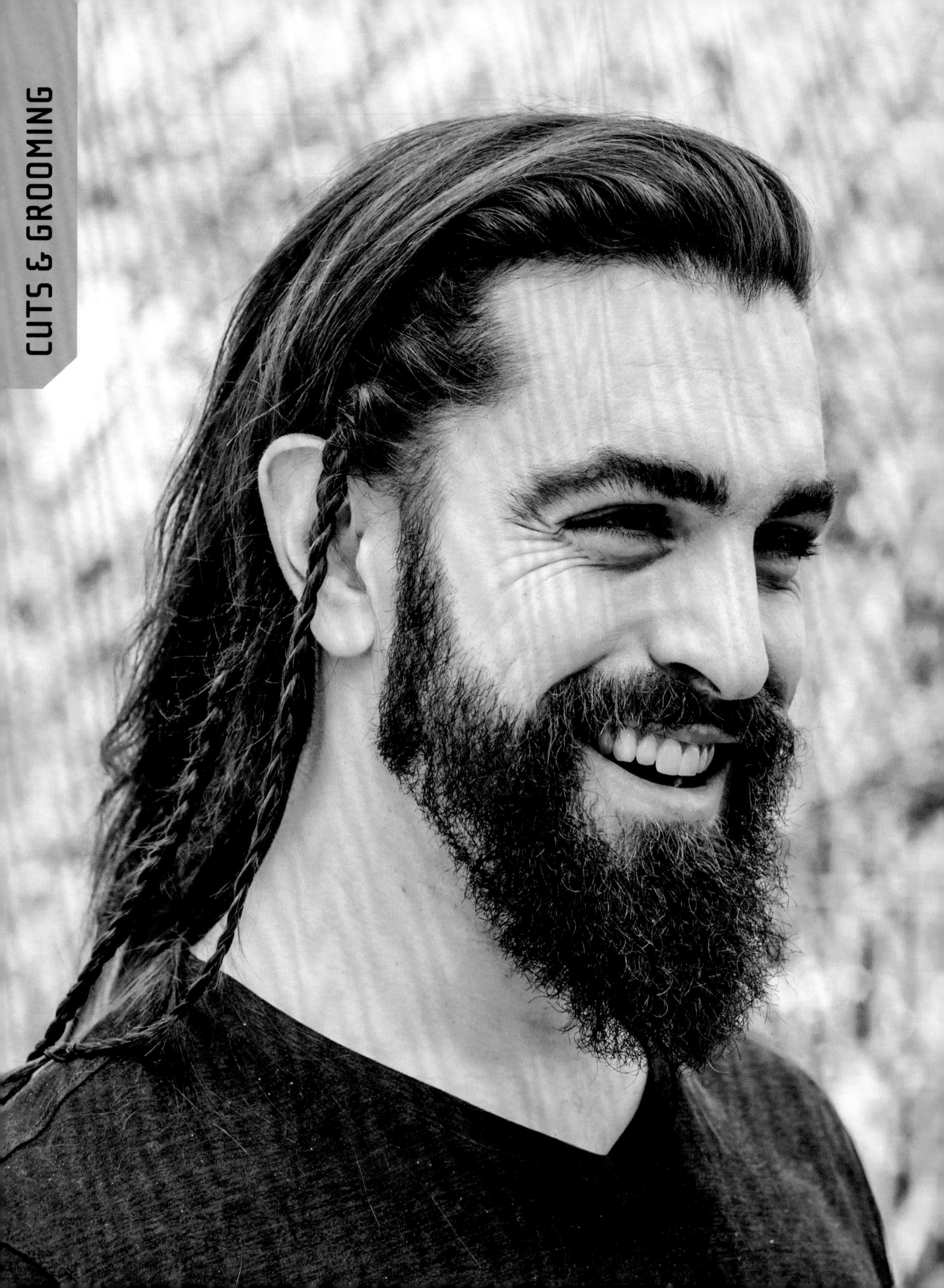

HAIR AND BEARD CARE

No matter how good you get at creating new looks for yourself, the basic condition of your hair will always be obvious. So, the better care you take of both the hair on your head and on your face, the better the end results will be once you start experimenting with styles.

WASHING

Wash your hair regularly to get rid of any added product (for most people, every two or three days is fine), but don't wash it too frequently or you will dry it out. Over-washing will strip the natural oils from your scalp, which are what keep hair looking shiny and healthy. Make sure that you select a shampoo designed for your hair type, and use conditioner if your hair needs it. Conditioner works by getting the scales down the hair shaft to lie flat, giving a shiny, smooth appearance.

DRYING

If you are using a hair dryer regularly—and I hope that you will be!—avoid using it for long stretches at a time, or always using it on the hottest setting. A hair dryer can dehydrate your hair, so try to let it dry naturally whenever you can to give it a break, or opt for a cool setting occasionally instead of a warm one to give your hair a gentler treatment. Hair is weaker when wet, too, so always use a comb rather than a brush on wet hair.

"SECOND-DAY" HAIR

Although it's good to clean your hair regularly, you will notice that it can actually be a lot easier to create certain styles with second-day hair. This is because freshly washed hair can be slippery and soft, making it harder to get it to do what you want. If you wait a day, you'll find that your hair will have a lot more natural hold and texture. And if your hair feels a bit greasy but not quite ready for washing, try a dry shampoo instead. These are a good interim measure, absorbing excess oils at the roots, and providing a bit of extra helpful volume.

BEARD CARE

It can be very easy to forget about the hair on your face, but once you start to use the products that I mention throughout Chapters 4 and 5, you will notice the difference.

A beard balm or oil will keep your beard supple and soft, while aftershave balm will keep the skin around it looking moisturized and fresh. Remember, too, that whatever beard or mustache you go for, it pays to maintain it, trimming when necessary. If your facial hair looks neat, the style will have much more impact.

FINDING A GOOD STYLIST

A stylist and a barber are two very different things—someone who styles your hair, as opposed to someone who cuts it—and although there are some who are good at both tasks, very often someone who is very skilled at cutting might not be so experienced when it comes to styling, and vice versa. So if you're looking for new ways to style the hair you already have—perhaps including a cut—then a hairdressing salon will probably be your best bet.

THE OVERALL PACKAGE

When it comes to deciding whether it's a stylist or a barber you're after, one of the key things is the experience you will have during your visit. If you want more of a laddish vibe, and a professional cut with clippers, then a barber is what you're after.

But you may prefer the atmosphere and level of customer service of a salon, where you will be able to consult hairstyle magazines, receive a full consultation, and be able to book an appointment in advance. Most hairdressers also offer a good selection of salon-quality products for sale, and will be able to advise you on exactly what to buy. A salon will usually be more expensive than a barber's, but it depends on what your priorities are.

Most hairdressers will do both men's and women's hair, but the majority of their customers will probably be women, so it's worth checking, and asking around for recommendations for a stylist who specializes in men's hair. (Although you can't generalize, either—I started out in hairdressing myself!)

VISUAL REFERENCES

When you go into a salon, it's really important to take a photo or two of what you want. This is the best way of communicating your wishes to your stylist. But do remember that you need to be realistic—your own hair's texture and shape, and your facial structure, may be completely different to the celeb in the shot. But as long as you take that into account, a photo of your desired style will definitely give your stylist a good starting point. And if they can't achieve the look, they will be able to explain why, and recommend something better for you.

TAKE-AWAY SKILLS

Make the most of your stylist's skills and ask them to teach you how to create the look yourself at home— ask them what products they've chosen, how and when they've applied them, and their method for blow-drying. Use your eyes, too. Watch them as they work, and then try to imitate their technique when you get home. You'll be the one styling your hair more than anyone else, so you have no excuses when it comes to being the expert on your own hair!

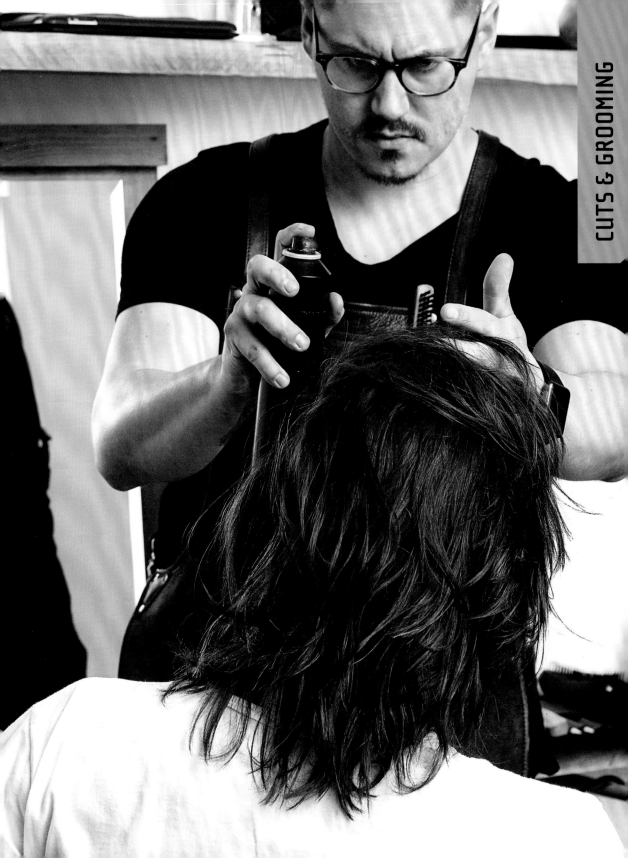

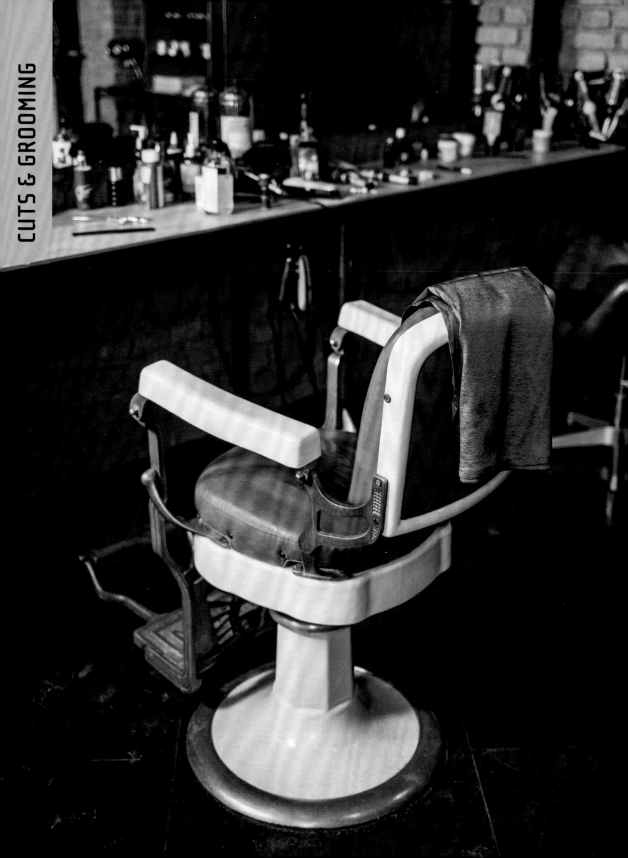

FINDING A GOOD BARBER

It sounds obvious, but make sure you always pick a barber who inspires complete confidence. Technique and skill really matter when it comes to a cut, because once it's gone there's nothing you can do until it grows back. And if your hair grows slowly, this is something you'll want to avoid. But on the other hand, don't avoid risk altogether—it's just hair, and sometimes you need to go out on a limb and try something new to know if it'll suit you!

CHEAP CUTS

Barbers are usually a lot cheaper than hairdressers, but the general rule of thumb in both cases is that you get what you pay for. The cheaper the cut, the faster they will work. You don't need to avoid walk-in barbershops, but it can be safer to go for one that costs just a little bit extra. A place offering quick cuts for $10 is usually going to be more concerned with plowing through a long queue of customers than offering you a personalized service. A good cut should really take around 30 to 45 minutes.

DO YOUR HOMEWORK

Today, there is a whole new breed of barbers out there offering a level of customer service to rival a hairdressing salon, alongside the old-school, traditional barbers, so it really pays to look around before you make your choice. This comes down to personal preference a lot of the time. Does the atmosphere make you feel comfortable? Is there good banter, and is the customer service slick and reassuring? Just because a barbershop looks nice isn't a guarantee, but it is definitely a sign that they care about what they do.

Hygiene can be another consideration. Do they have Barbicide disinfectant jars out on display, for example? Do they spray their clippers with Clippercide between cuts? These things matter.

TAKE A VISUAL

As when visiting a stylist, take a picture of what you have in mind when you visit a barber. That way they'll be clear on what you want right from the start. If they're skilled and experienced, they'll also be able to advise you of any potential issues—what will and won't be achievable with your hair type and face shape.

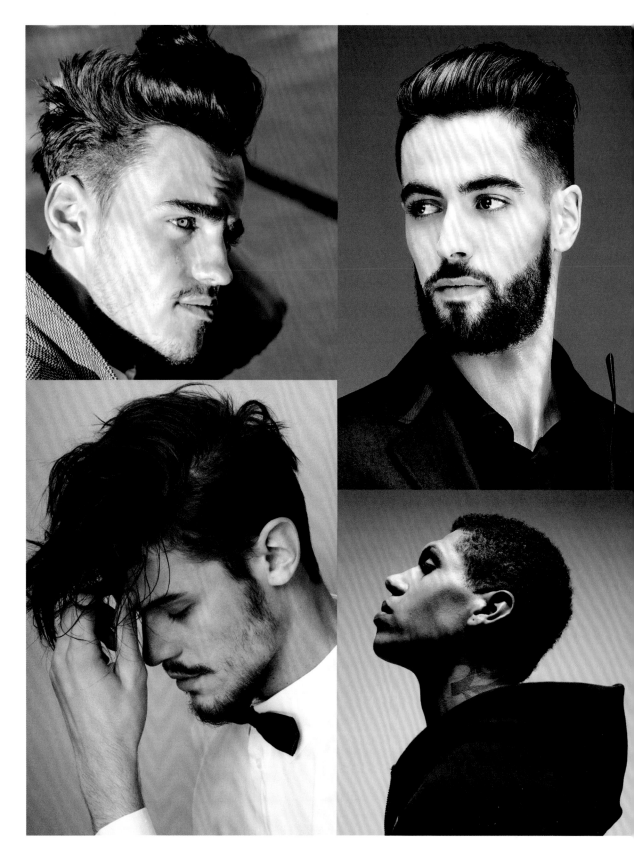

CHAPTER 2

TEXTURED QUIFF

If you have the right sort of hair for this look, then I guarantee it will end up becoming one of your go-to styles because it's so versatile. It can be worn with pretty much anything—formal or casual—so it's great for going straight from work to a night out. I've kept the process nice and easy, too, by towel-drying rather than using a hair dryer.

DIFFICULTY – Easy

IDEAL FACE SHAPE – All shapes, but not too triangular

IDEAL HAIR – Sleek, straight hair

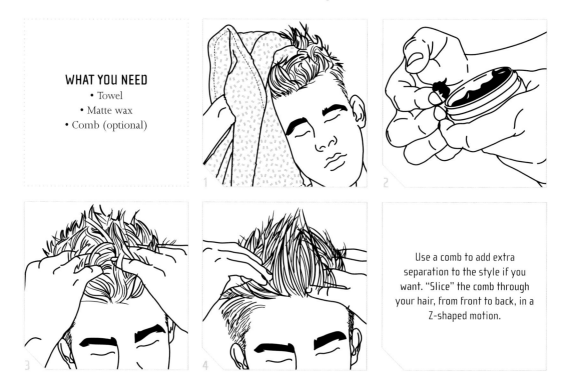

WHAT YOU NEED
- Towel
- Matte wax
- Comb (optional)

Use a comb to add extra separation to the style if you want. "Slice" the comb through your hair, from front to back, in a Z-shaped motion.

1. Start with wet hair, and begin by towel-drying it thoroughly, getting it as dry as you can all over before moving to the next step.

2. Now take a portion of matte wax and rub it between your fingers.

3. Next, apply the wax everywhere with your fingers, making sure you distribute it evenly throughout your hair.

4. Finish off by defining the quiff using your fingers, as shown.

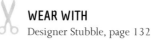

WEAR WITH
Designer Stubble, page 132

TOP TIP

Experiment with the quantity of wax you use. Too little will not provide sufficient hold, and too much will weigh your hair down.

TOP TIP

Make life easier by buying a comb that has wide teeth at one end, and small teeth at the other.

SUPERMAN SIDE PART

A Clark Kent side part is an enduring style that somehow manages to look both retro and modern. It also suits anyone. Do note, though, that if you have a round face, you should avoid making it too flat; and if you have a long face, you don't want to create too much height or you'll elongate your face.

DIFFICULTY – Easy

IDEAL FACE SHAPE – All shapes

IDEAL HAIR – Straight, textured, or wavy hair—less effective on curly hair

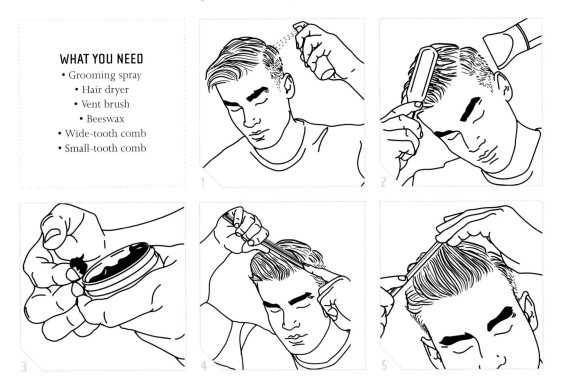

WHAT YOU NEED
- Grooming spray
- Hair dryer
- Vent brush
- Beeswax
- Wide-tooth comb
- Small-tooth comb

1. Apply your choice of grooming spray to your hair while wet. This can be anything that will provide both hold and volume, so experiment to find the product that suits you best.

2. Now blow-dry your hair in the right direction, starting at the part. Use your vent brush to lift the hair and hold it over to one side, while directing the air down on the hair. Unlike the Soft Side Part (page 48), you need to keep this flat and sleek.

3. For plenty of shine, I've used beeswax as my finishing product. Grab a dime-sized amount and work it between your fingers before running it evenly through your hair.

4. Now use your small-tooth comb to create a clean and decisive part.

5. Then use your wide-tooth comb to comb your hair neatly into place, away from the part.

 WEAR WITH
Clean Shave, page 144

MESSY BEDHEAD

The clue with this look is in the name. Since you want to look like you just rolled out of bed, the messier this is, the better! It's another style that you can really enjoy creating because, although you start with a hair dryer, you don't need to be too fussy about technique. Simply focus on giving your hair as much texture as possible.

DIFFICULTY - Medium
IDEAL FACE SHAPE - All face shapes
IDEAL HAIR - Sleek and straight

WHAT YOU NEED
- Hair dryer
- Flat iron
- Matte wax

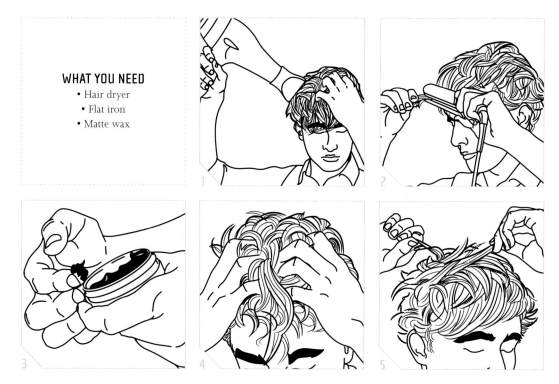

1. With your hair washed but still wet, begin by giving it a thorough blast with your hair dryer.

2. Now use the flat iron to straighten out small sections of hair. Clamp the iron over the hair, and then slide it up, working from the roots to the ends with each new section.

3. Next, take a dab of matte wax and work it between your fingers.

4. Add the wax to your hair and work it through thoroughly, moving from front to back, left to right—every which way—keeping it all nice and messy. Push your hair up into the center, too.

5. Finish off by picking out small tufts of hair and tugging them in different directions to add texture.

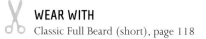

WEAR WITH
Classic Full Beard (short), page 118

TOP TIP

Matte wax does double duty for this style—providing hold as well as a sufficiently lived-in matte texture.

TOP TIP

If you start with wet hair you'll find it easier to make your hair sit in the direction you want.

CLASSIC POMPADOUR

As I've mentioned, in my experience most guys hate using a hair dyer—but to get the volume you require for this look, you will need to overcome your fears! (As with several styles in this book, the need for a dryer is the only reason I've rated this style "medium" in terms of difficulty.) This looks good on anyone, but if you've got a long face, just don't let the pomp get too high.

DIFFICULTY – Medium

IDEAL FACE SHAPE – All face shapes

IDEAL HAIR – Straight, curly, or wavy

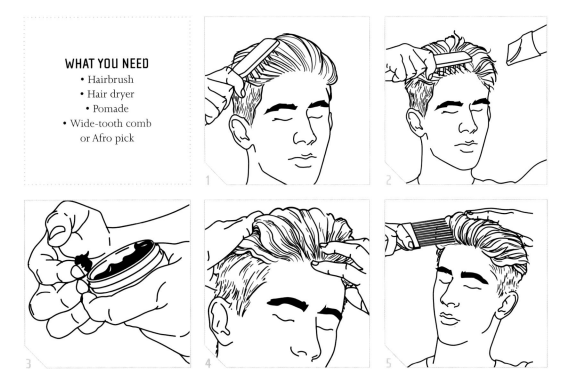

WHAT YOU NEED
- Hairbrush
- Hair dryer
- Pomade
- Wide-tooth comb or Afro pick

1. Start with wet hair, and brush it toward the back of your head.

2. Now, using your hair dryer, dry your hair and prime it ready for product. Make sure you hold the dryer higher than your brush and at an angle, so that the airflow travels along the hair shaft, keeping the hair cuticle flat. This will keep your hair smooth and sleek.

3. Scoop out a dime-sized portion of pomade and rub it between your fingers.

4. Now apply the product to your hair, raking it through evenly and thoroughly with your fingers.

5. Finally, work your pick or comb gently through your hair, sweeping it in the right direction without losing any of the volume that you've built up.

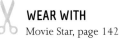

WEAR WITH
Movie Star, page 142

MODERN POMPADOUR

This style is very similar to a classic "pomp" (page 42), but rather than having everything swept neatly back off the face for a streamlined, perfected finish in the traditional way, this version has a much softer, looser feel. This modern take on a classic uses the same techniques as the original, but produces a more adaptable style.

DIFFICULTY – Medium

IDEAL FACE SHAPE – All face shapes

IDEAL HAIR – Slick or wavy

WHAT YOU NEED
- Volumizing or texture spray
- Hair dryer
- Flat brush
- Pomade
- Comb

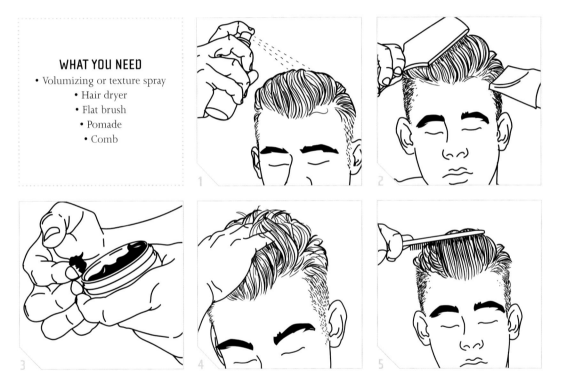

1. Start by spritzing your wet hair with the volumizing or texturizing spray product of your choice. When choosing a volumizing product, take into account how much volume you want to create, and how much hold your hair requires.

2. Now blow-dry your hair into shape, sweeping it back as you go by using a flat brush, as shown.

3. When your hair is dry, scoop out a small dollop of pomade and warm it up between your fingers.

4. Now work the product through your hair thoroughly, raking it through with your fingers from front to back. When it has been distributed throughout, create a smooth finish by running an open hand over your hair.

5. The final touch is to sweep your comb back through your hair to add volume, definition, and impact.

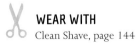

WEAR WITH
Clean Shave, page 144

TOP TIP

Slick hair tends to need a bit more product than hair that naturally has some texture to it.

TOP TIP

I've used a mattifying wax for the look shown here, but you could substitute a beeswax product for more shine and a softer feel.

BIG-VOLUME QUIFF

This style is perfect if you want to give your hair a dramatic retro edge. It's versatile, too—you can pair it with anything from a high-fashion suit to a casual combination of T-shirt, jeans, and jacket. Since I've kept this simple and created the look without a brush, you'll be at an advantage if your hair already has a bit of texture to it.

DIFFICULTY - Medium

IDEAL FACE SHAPE - All faces, though it would elongate an already-long face

IDEAL HAIR - Straight to wavy

WHAT YOU NEED
- Spray volumizing product
- Hair dryer
- Matte wax
- Hairspray

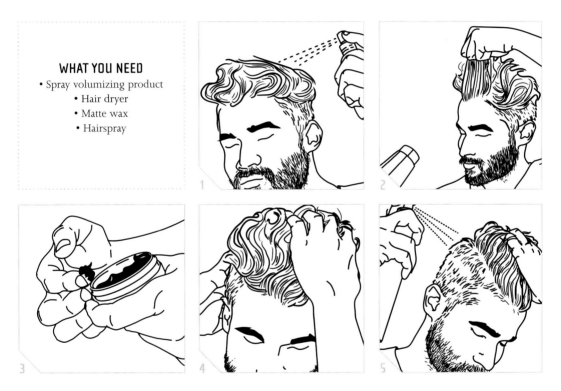

1. Start with wet hair and apply your chosen volumizing product, holding the applicator about 8 inches (20 cm) away from your hair.

2. With your hair dryer, start building up some volume using your hands. Remove the nozzle from the dryer for maximum volume. (If you want a smoother effect, though, keep the nozzle in place—it will direct the air flow and create less "disturbance.")

3. Next, scoop out a tiny portion of wax, then warm it up between your fingers.

4. Run your fingers through your hair, sweeping them in the direction that you want your hair to sit.

5. Finish off by applying a bit of hairspray to give the style extra hold throughout the day.

 WEAR WITH
Handlebar 'Tache, page 158

SOFT SIDE PART

This is another easy part to achieve—similar to the Superman Side Part (page 38), but looser, softer, and more casual. It works well for most hair types, apart from curly hair. Curly hair can be slicked back without any problems, but it often can't be made to sit softly—it's all too easy to end up with just a big lump of hair on one side!

DIFFICULTY - Medium

IDEAL FACE SHAPE - All shapes

IDEAL HAIR - All hair types—less effective with curly hair

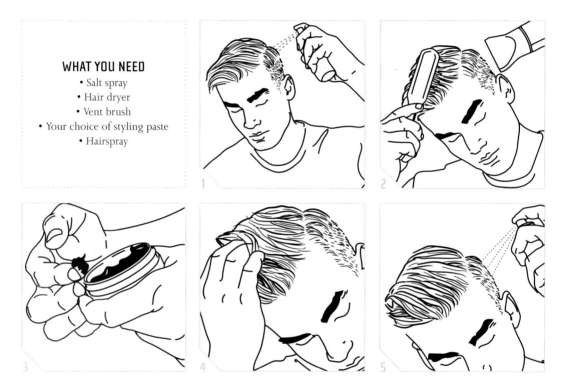

WHAT YOU NEED
- Salt spray
- Hair dryer
- Vent brush
- Your choice of styling paste
- Hairspray

1. Apply your choice of grooming spray to your hair while it's still wet. I've used a salt spray here, but you can use whatever you like, depending on the hold, texture, and volume you want.

2. Now use your hair dryer to dry your hair and add a bit of volume at the same time. Do this by using your vent brush to lift up the hair at the roots, at the part, and then hold it over to the desired side, while directing your dryer down onto it, as shown.

3. Next, grab a small dab of styling paste (you could use pomade, fiber paste, or a styling cream) and work it between your fingers.

4. Then use your hands to sweep it through your hair, making sure that you work in the right direction.

5. Finish off with an application of hairspray.

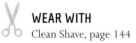

WEAR WITH
Clean Shave, page 144

TOP TIP

Get good at using your fingers to
tweak the ends in order to create
exactly the texture and shape
that suits you.

TOP TIP

The best hair for this style is dead straight, so if you have wavy hair, use a flat iron to straighten it first (page 76).

TWISTS

This is a style to have fun with. As with the Spiky Texture look on page 78, you apply a product to your hair, then work random sections for the desired finished look. Here, though, you twist each section, creating as few or as many twists as you like. I used a strong-hold matte wax on my model, but substitute beeswax if you want more shine.

DIFFICULTY – Medium
IDEAL FACE SHAPE – All face shapes
IDEAL HAIR – Straight, short hair

WHAT YOU NEED
- Hair dryer
- Matte wax or beeswax
- Hairspray
- Flat iron (optional)

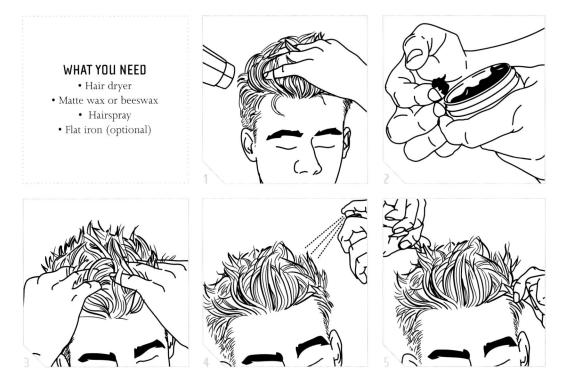

1. Start by rough-drying your hair with your hair dryer and your hands to give it a bit of extra texture before you begin styling it.

2. Now take a portion of matte wax and rub it between your fingers.

3. Apply the product throughout your hair with your fingers, making sure you distribute it evenly.

4. Next, apply some hairspray all over, which will give the style additional hold, especially if you have slightly longer hair.

5. Finish off by creating twists with your fingers, as shown. Focus on small sections all over the top of your head and around your face to create the desired look.

 WEAR WITH
Designer Stubble, page 132

SLICKBACK

The difficulty level of this timeless style depends more on the nature of your hair than your skill level. If you have unruly hair, you'll need to start with it wet, and then use a hair dryer and a flat brush to sweep it back flat. But if your hair stays in place by itself, then you may find that using product alone will be enough.

DIFFICULTY – Easy to medium
IDEAL FACE SHAPE – All shapes
IDEAL HAIR – Straight, wavy, but not curly

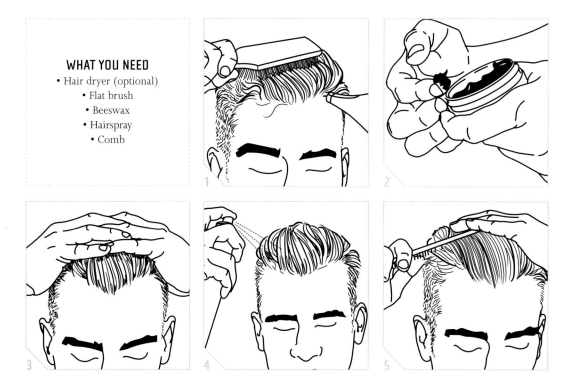

WHAT YOU NEED
- Hair dryer (optional)
- Flat brush
- Beeswax
- Hairspray
- Comb

1. Start with wet hair and blow-dry it back, using your flat brush to guide the direction, as shown.

2. Now take a bit of beeswax and rub it between your fingers. Don't go crazy with it—you can always add more if you need to!

3. Now sweep the beeswax through your hair, running your flat palms over it from front to back to create a smooth, sleek appearance.

4. Give your hair a quick spritz of hairspray all over. The beeswax will provide shine, but you'll need the hairspray to give you extra hold.

5. Then finish off by slicking everything back neatly with your comb.

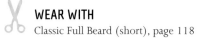

WEAR WITH
Classic Full Beard (short), page 118

TOP TIP

Always blow-dry in the direction that you want the hair to sit —from the front to the back.

TOP TIP

Oil sheen sprays are great for curly hair. They don't add volume, but they seal your hair, defining curls and preventing frizz.

CURLY TEXTURE

Even if you have the right hair type for this casual style, it is worth assessing what your hair needs in terms of product. If it's very curly, hold will be less of an issue, but you'll need hydration: a curl cream, a serum—anything that seals the cuticle and adds moisture. My model had naturally looser curls to begin with, so I chose fiber paste, which tames frizz but also provides hold and definition.

DIFFICULTY - Medium

IDEAL FACE SHAPE - All face shapes

IDEAL HAIR - Wavy and curly hair only

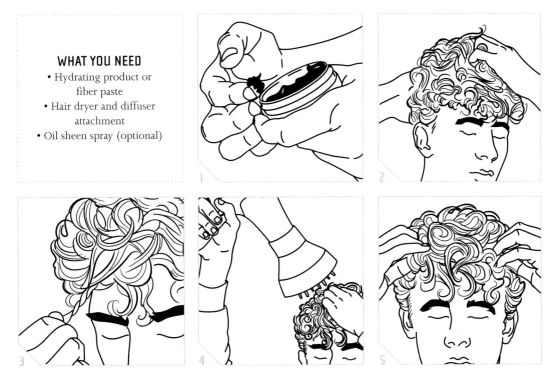

WHAT YOU NEED
- Hydrating product or fiber paste
- Hair dryer and diffuser attachment
- Oil sheen spray (optional)

1. Start with wet hair. Take a small amount of your chosen product and warm it between your fingers.

2. Work the product through your hair, scrunching it with your hands to create a bit of body.

3. Now start twisting random small sections of hair to create extra interest and texture. If your hair is very long, you can twist some strands around a finger to really define the curl.

4. Now dry your hair using your hair dryer, with its diffuser attachment in place. This will provide heat

without a strong airflow, preventing your hair from getting too frizzy, which is often an issue with curly hair. Keep working your hair gently with your hands to keep the movement in it.

5. Once dry, reapply a bit more of your chosen product for extra definition and hold where needed.

 WEAR WITH
Petite Goatee, page 136

AFRO SPONGE

For this style I'm using a double-sided curl or twist sponge—with evenly spaced small holes on one side and wavy foam spikes on the other side—which gives you two different styling options in one simple tool, achievable in just minutes. Although this type of sponge doesn't last forever, they can be purchased very cheaply, so make sure that you replace it when it starts to get worn out.

DIFFICULTY – Easy

IDEAL FACE SHAPE – All face shapes

IDEAL HAIR – Afro

WHAT YOU NEED
- Olive oil spray or similar sheen spray
- Grooming cream
- Double-sided curl sponge

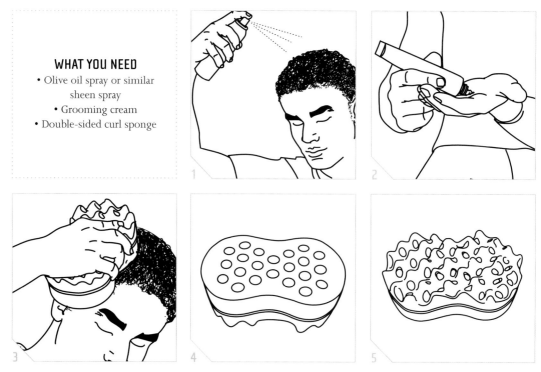

1. Begin by spraying your dry hair with an olive oil spray or similar, so that it is soft, supple, and moisturized before you begin.

2. Now take a small amount of grooming cream, work it between your fingers, and then scrunch it through your hair, distributing it evenly all over.

3. Next, work the sponge against your head, using small circular motions, and working all over your head. Use the sponge side of your choice, depending on the effect you want (see Steps 4 and 5) and always work in one direction only—clockwise or counterclockwise.

4. The little holes on one side of the sponge will make smaller, tighter coils.

5. The protrusions on the other side of the sponge will make looser coils with more volume.

WEAR WITH
Designer Stubble, page 132

TOP TIP

Only apply light pressure with the sponge—you do not need to press hard to get results.

TOP TIP

If you want to keep this look fixed in place all day, use a firm-hold hairspray after styling.

TEXTURED CROP

This is a very current look that is also very easy to create and maintain. It's perfect for giving emphasis to strong features. It does suit most face shapes, too, although if your face is very round it might not be the perfect choice as it will only exaggerate this.

DIFFICULTY – Easy

IDEAL FACE SHAPE – Oval, square, heart-shaped—less suited to round faces

IDEAL HAIR – Sleek or wavy

WHAT YOU NEED
- Towel
- Matte wax
- Firm-hold hairspray (optional)
- Flat iron (optional)

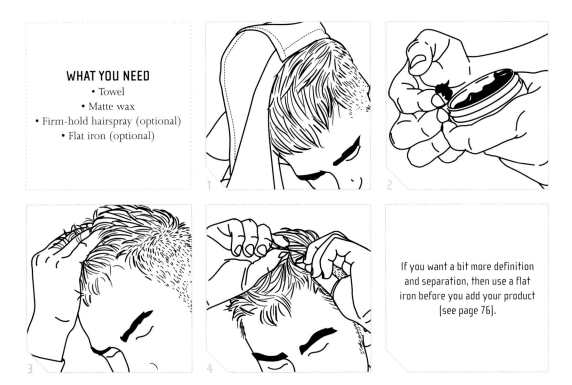

If you want a bit more definition and separation, then use a flat iron before you add your product (see page 76).

1. Start with wet hair, and begin by toweling it dry as thoroughly as you can.

2. Now grab a tiny bit of matte wax and warm it up between your fingers. The shorter your hair is, the less you will need.

3. Work the wax into your hair with your fingers, raking it through, scrunching it—doing whatever it takes to distribute it evenly and also get plenty of shape and texture. My model here has very short sides, so I mostly applied wax to the longer hair on top.

4. Finish off by "piecing" your style. This involves adding texture by separating out small random sections of hair and working them between your fingers.

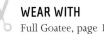

WEAR WITH
Full Goatee, page 134

PERFECT AFRO

If you're lucky enough to have Afro hair then you have the potential for amazing styles with very little effort. But that doesn't mean you can skip the basics—it's still important to keep your hair well moisturized and combed. A pick is the perfect tool for combing your hair; its long, thin teeth reach right down into the roots without disrupting the texture and volume of the hair above.

DIFFICULTY - Easy

IDEAL FACE SHAPE - All shapes

IDEAL HAIR - Afro

WHAT YOU NEED
• Olive oil spray or other sheen spray
• Grooming cream
• Afro pick
• Boar-bristle brush

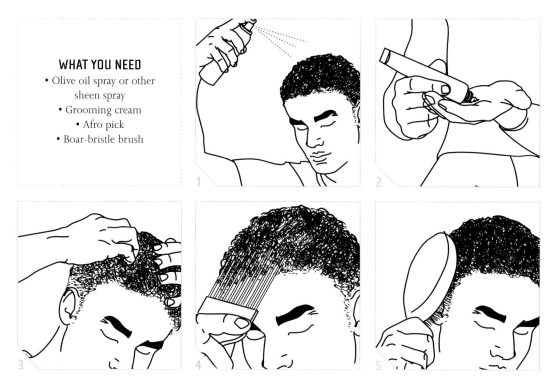

1. Begin by spraying your hair with an olive oil spray or similar, to make it soft and supple.

2. Now take a small amount of grooming cream and work it between your fingers.

3. Work the cream through your hair, scrunching your hair with your fingers.

4. Now use a pick to work through your hair in sections at a time, getting rid of tangles and gently

lifting the hair at the roots. The long teeth of the pick should allow you to work without disrupting the volume you've built up.

5. When you are done with the pick, finish off by using a boar-bristle brush on the sides to keep them neat and flat.

WEAR WITH

Petite Goatee, page 136

TOP TIP

Work the pick all over the head in different directions to ensure maximum volume.

TOP TIP

Using a brush while hair-drying will give you greater control and direction.

SLICK UNDERCUT

An undercut is essentially a style that is shorter underneath, but kept longer on top, with a clear definition between these two areas. But within this category you will see lots of different length and contrast variations. My model here has been clipped short at the sides, with quite a bit of length left on top, which gives plenty of options for styling.

DIFFICULTY – Medium

IDEAL FACE SHAPE – All shapes

IDEAL HAIR – Good for straight, wavy, or curly hair

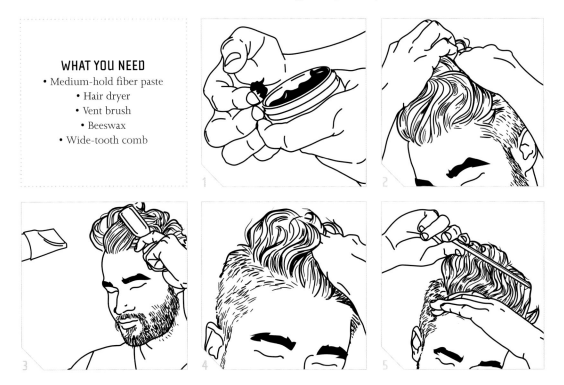

WHAT YOU NEED
- Medium-hold fiber paste
- Hair dryer
- Vent brush
- Beeswax
- Wide-tooth comb

1. Start with wet hair. Grab a tiny bit of paste from the pot and rub it together it between your fingers.

2. Now run the fiber paste evenly through your hair with your fingers, sweeping your hair back in the right direction.

3. Next, blow-dry your hair, slicking everything to one side as you go, using your brush.

4. You will now need to apply a small quantity of beeswax to give the look a bit of a sheen, working it through the top and sides of your hair using your hands.

5. Finish off by combing through the style, shaping it with your fingers as you go.

WEAR WITH
Sideburns, page 150

MID-LENGTH MOVEMENT

As the name suggests, this style is all about getting movement in your hair, using a combination of hands, product, brush, and dryer. The more you practice, the better you'll get, so stick with it. The trick is to respect the natural texture and shape of your hair. So if you have any kinks or a cowlick, for example, don't fight them—make the most of them.

DIFFICULTY – Medium

IDEAL FACE SHAPE – All face shapes

IDEAL HAIR – Straight through to wavy, but trickier with curly hair

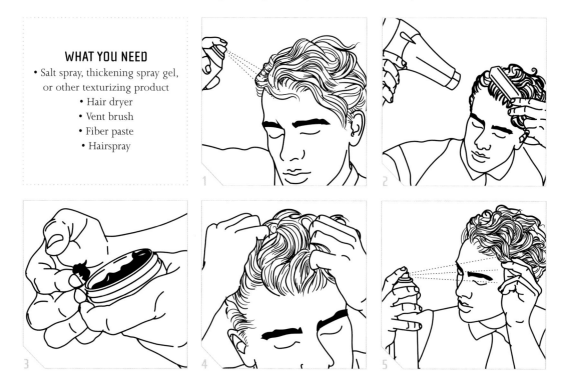

WHAT YOU NEED
- Salt spray, thickening spray gel, or other texturizing product
- Hair dryer
- Vent brush
- Fiber paste
- Hairspray

1. Start by applying your choice of texturizing product to freshly washed hair. You can use salt spray, thickening spray gel, or anything that gives it a second-day feel and hold.

2. Now blow it dry using your hair dryer and a vent brush, sweeping it back and to one side.

3. Grab a small portion of fiber paste and warm it up between your fingers.

4. Apply the paste to your hair, scrunching it in all over. This will add further definition and will also help to hold the shape of the style in place.

5. Finally, set the finished look with a light mist of hairspray, holding the can about 8 inches (20 cm) from your hair.

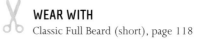

WEAR WITH
Classic Full Beard (short), page 118

TOP TIP

Wavy hair won't need too much
fiber paste; on straight hair,
apply more, but in stages,
building up the shape gradually.

TOP TIP

Medium-hold fiber paste suits finer hair, whereas matte wax suits thicker hair.

SLEEK CROP

When it comes to bangs, some guys like to cut them all off, or keep them swept away
from their face. But this military-esque style is for those who want to wear them down
and make them work with their face shape. It's all about adding movement,
and creating variation with what otherwise might be a simple haircut.

DIFFICULTY – Medium

IDEAL FACE SHAPE – Most shapes, but suits strong features

IDEAL HAIR – Straight hair

WHAT YOU NEED
- Hair dryer
- Flat brush
- Fiber paste or matte wax, depending on hair texture
- Medium-hold hairspray

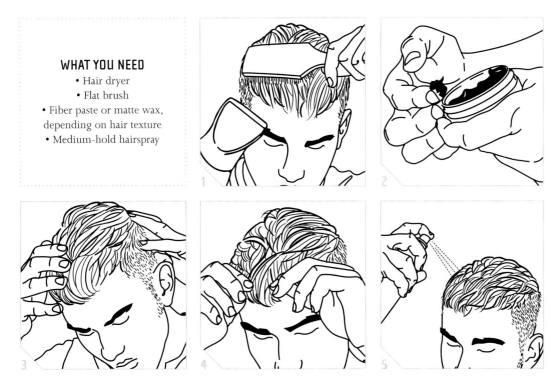

1. Start by drying your wet hair with your hair dryer and flat brush. Dry from the back to the front, and then from side to side, "dragging" your hair across with the brush and directing the air flow to follow in the same direction. This will keep the hair cuticle lying flat and smooth.

2. Take a small amount of your chosen product and work it between your fingers.

3. Now run the product through your hair, again working from the back to front, and from side to side, sweeping your hair in the desired direction.

4. Then, using your fingers, scrunch texture into your fringe until you have the desired effect.

5. Finish off with some hairpsray to hold everything in place, from about 8 inches (20 cm) away, aiming it down from above and avoiding your eyes.

WEAR WITH
Full Goatee, page 134

CURLY HALO

This is one for the curly haired, but that doesn't mean you can do without using product! I've actually used two different products here—a curl cream to enhance the curl and hydrate the hair, and then a fiber paste to hold the curl in place. If your hair still doesn't curl up well, don't be afraid to use a bit of mousse before hair-drying, too.

DIFFICULTY - Medium

IDEAL FACE SHAPE - Oval, square, or triangular

IDEAL HAIR - Wavy to curly

WHAT YOU NEED
- Curl cream
- Hair dryer
- Fiber paste
- Hairspray

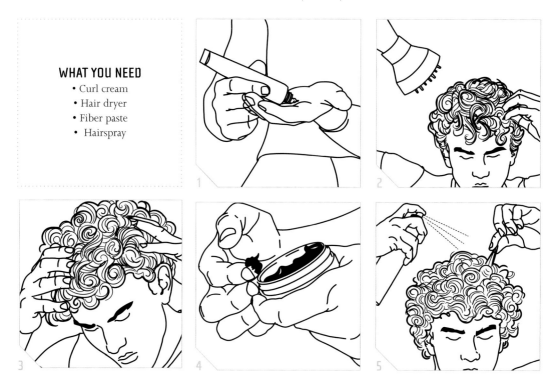

1. Start with wet hair. Take a bit of curl cream in your hands and rub it between your palms.

2. Use the diffuser attachment on your hair dryer to blow-dry your hair, scrunching your hair with your hands as you work.

3. Now shake your hair out, moving your hands back and forth to get maximum movement in it.

4. Grab a small portion of fiber paste with a finger and then work it between your palms. You then need to

apply this to your hair using a "scrunching" motion, grabbing chunks of hair at a time.

5. Spray with hairspray, while pulling out a few random small strands to add detail and texture.

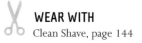

WEAR WITH
Clean Shave, page 144

TOP TIP

If your hair is not as curly as you'd like, use mousse and make extra twists with your fingers before blow-drying.

TOP TIP

The texturizing spray and matte wax should be enough for this style, but if your hair is very thick and heavy, you may want to finish with a bit of hairspray.

MODERN ROCK 'N' ROLLER

Guys in the '50s would have worn this style all the time, and it's making a real comeback.
What I've created here is a modern rock 'n' roller—tons of height and volume at the front,
with the sides left quite short. The only hair type that this style doesn't work for is curly hair,
since you'd have to work against your natural texture to get the right shape.

DIFFICULTY – Medium

IDEAL FACE SHAPE – All face shapes

IDEAL HAIR – Straight to wavy—not curly

WHAT YOU NEED
- Texturizing spray
- Flat brush
- Hair dryer
- Matte wax
- Hairspray (optional)

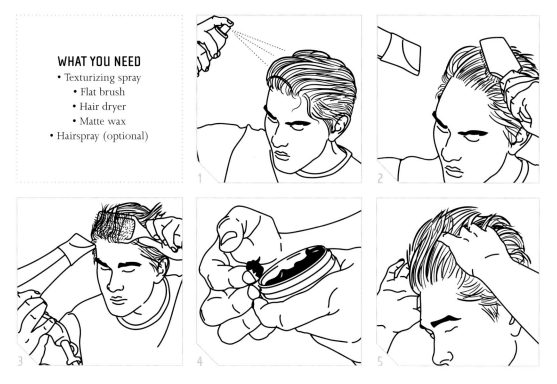

1. Begin by applying texturizing spray to wet hair, getting overall coverage for sufficient hold.

2. Now blow-dry your hair with the aid of a flat brush, establishing the basic shape of the style.

3. For volume at the front, dry from the roots up to the ends. You need to use a "forward and upward" motion with your brush and dryer to set the shape in place—hold the hair forward with your brush to begin with, then swoop it back in a wave shape, keeping the dryer hovering over each section as you work.

4. Now warm up a bit of wax between your fingers.

5. Finish by sweeping it back through your hair, first to one side, and then the other, for even distribution, without losing any of the height you've built up at the front.

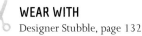

WEAR WITH
Designer Stubble, page 132

ELEPHANT'S TRUNK

This is essentially a modern take on a classic rock 'n' roll hairstyle that Teddy Boys used to wear—the traditional version was usually created on hair that was an inch or two longer than my model's hair. It has a similar length and style to a pomp (see page 42), but here you blow-dry your hair so that it sits forward.

DIFFICULTY – Medium to hard

IDEAL FACE SHAPE – All shapes

IDEAL HAIR – Straight, wavy, or curly

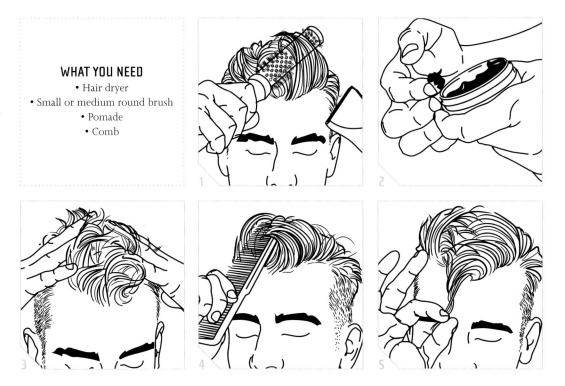

WHAT YOU NEED
- Hair dryer
- Small or medium round brush
- Pomade
- Comb

1. Starting with wet hair, you will begin by building up the basic shape of this style with your hair dryer. Take a small section of your hair and curl it around your round brush, as shown. Then use your hair dryer to dry it in place, wrapped around the brush.

2. Now grab a dime-sized portion of pomade and distribute it between your fingers.

3. Sweep the product through your hair, working from the back to the front, and pushing your hair up into a peak at the center at the same time.

4. Now perfect the shape at the front with your comb, gently twisting the hair into the elephant's trunk.

5. Then, to finish off the style, twist the end of the trunk with your fingers to create a final bit of curl and definition.

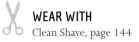

WEAR WITH
Clean Shave, page 144

TOP TIP

The hair dryer and brush do a lot of the work for you with this style, so practice your technique as often as you can.

TOP TIP

Using a comb after you have applied your beeswax and not before gives maximum definition.

MID-LENGTH SLICKBACK

When using a hair dryer, always work toward the result you are trying to achieve. For a slickback that sits fairly close to your head, pull sections of hair taut with the brush as you dry them—to the back, over to one side, and then the other—for a flat, smooth finish. My model's hair is naturally wavy, so his slickback has a lot of body, but if your hair is straight, you'll get a much flatter, slicker result.

DIFFICULTY - Medium

IDEAL FACE SHAPE - All face shapes

IDEAL HAIR - Best on sleek or wavy hair; less effective on curly hair

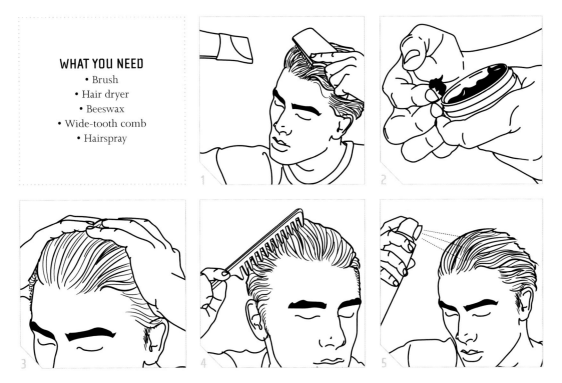

WHAT YOU NEED
- Brush
- Hair dryer
- Beeswax
- Wide-tooth comb
- Hairspray

1. Starting with wet hair, begin creating your desired shape by blow-drying your hair while sweeping it back with your brush. Making it nice and sleek at this stage will help with styling later.

2. Now take a small portion of beeswax and work it between your fingers.

3. Apply the beeswax to your hair, running your fingers through the strands and working from front to back, then passing the flats of your hands over it.

4. Next, sweep your hair back into position with your comb, creating a neat, smooth finish.

5. A spritz of hairspray should then hold it all in place for hours.

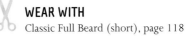

WEAR WITH
Classic Full Beard (short), page 118

TEXTURED UNDERCUT

It's important with an undercut (see also Slick Undercut, page 62) that the "disconnection"—
the difference in length between top and bottom—is at least an inch. The top needs to be
longer by this amount so that the visual difference between the two areas is obvious.
For this style you'll also be using a new tool—a flat iron.

DIFFICULTY - Medium

IDEAL FACE SHAPE - All shapes

IDEAL HAIR - All hair textures, though less effective on Afro hair

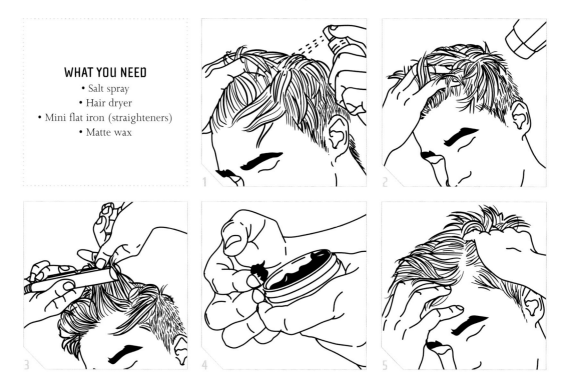

WHAT YOU NEED
- Salt spray
- Hair dryer
- Mini flat iron (straighteners)
- Matte wax

1. Start by adding salt spray to wet hair. This gives a nice rough, lived-in texture, and will make your hair much easier to mold and style.

2. Now roughly dry your hair with your hair dryer, tousling sections of it by hand as you direct the airflow.

3. You are now ready for the flat iron. Trust me, this is not something to fear! Simply hold up a section of hair and clamp it in the iron at the roots, as shown. Now move the iron steadily up the hair, traveling from the roots to the ends. The heat will flatten the hair cuticle and add texture. I am using a mini iron here, but you can also use a standard-sized iron.

4. Warm up a bit of wax between your fingers.

5. Run your fingers through your hair, moving all over, and in all directions, to create maximum texture.

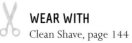

WEAR WITH
Clean Shave, page 144

TOP TIP

When using the flat iron, don't go over the same piece repeatedly or it will damage the hair.

TOP TIP

For extra definition, use your comb to pluck out small bits and pieces randomly.

SPIKY TEXTURE

This is a style that calls for a bit of creativity, and no two versions will be the same. The idea is to make it as messy as you like, taking advantage of the texture that you've created in the first couple of steps, and pulling your hair in all directions. It does need a hair dryer, but when you find out how easy this is, that won't put you off—and even the comb is optional!

DIFFICULTY - Medium

IDEAL FACE SHAPE - All face shapes

IDEAL HAIR - All types

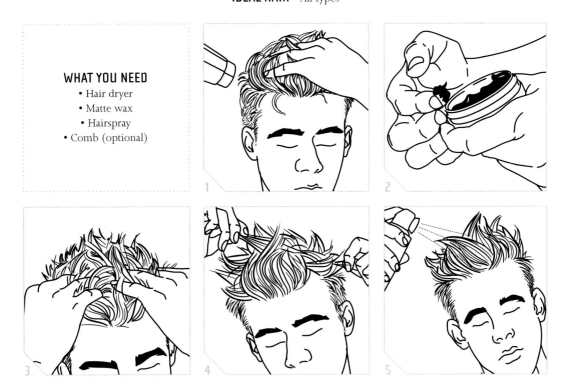

WHAT YOU NEED
- Hair dryer
- Matte wax
- Hairspray
- Comb (optional)

1. Start by rough-drying your hair with your hair dryer and your hands to create a bit of rough texture right from the start.

2. Now take a portion of matte wax and rub it between your fingers.

3. Apply the product throughout your hair with your fingers, working from the roots to the tips.

4. Now concentrate on creating as much mad, messy texture as you can, using your fingers. Pull sections of hair in random, opposing directions to get it looking as wild as you can.

5. Finally, give it all a blast of hairspray to set the style for the day—or night!

WEAR WITH
Designer Stubble, page 132

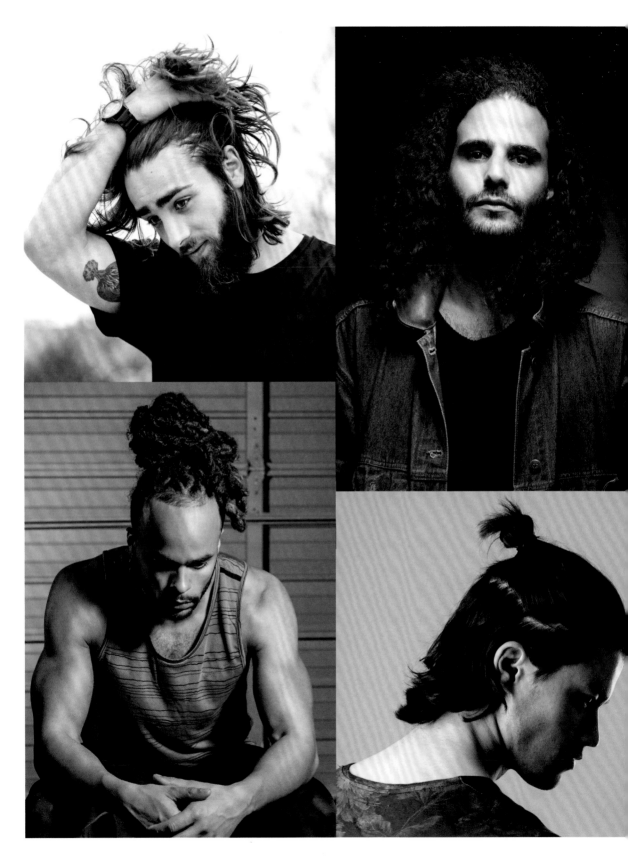

CHAPTER 3

BEACH WAVES

There are no prizes for guessing what the aim is with this casual style—hair that looks like you've just spent the day at the beach! Salt spray and fiber paste are the perfect combination for achieving this. You don't want to look completely windswept, but you do need to mimic the texture that sand and sea would naturally give your hair. I've classified this as a short style, but you will need a bit of length in your hair.

DIFFICULTY – Medium

IDEAL FACE SHAPE – All shapes

IDEAL HAIR – Straight to wavy hair

WHAT YOU NEED
- Salt spray
- Hair dryer
- Fiber paste
- Hairspray

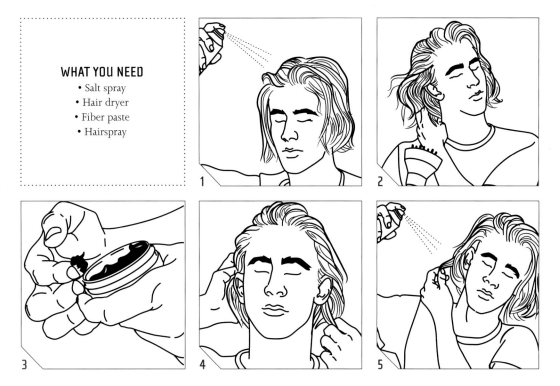

1. Start by giving your hair a thorough spritzing with the salt spray.

2. Now blow-dry your hair with the dryer's diffuser attachment in place. The warmth of the air will dry your hair without introducing any extra volume.

3. Grab a dime-size portion of fiber paste and warm it up between your fingers.

4. Run the paste through your hair, building up the texture and messiness.

5. And finally, a light application of hairspray will lock in all the product layers, preserving the style for hours.

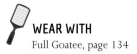

WEAR WITH
Full Goatee, page 134

TOP TIP

Don't introduce extra volume with the hair dryer; just "cement" in the effect of the salt spray for a natural-looking texture.

TOP TIP

Tugging at the edges of the finished braid will loosen it up a bit, but be careful not to dislodge your work. Tug evenly along the length of the braid on both sides.

BRAIDED PONY

Brace yourself—for this style you are going to have to learn to do a three-strand braid. This is the simplest braid there is, so even if this braid sits at the back of your head, it's really just a matter of following the instructions, step by step. Failing that, just pray and hope for the best!

DIFFICULTY - Medium

IDEAL FACE SHAPE - All face shapes

IDEAL HAIR - All textures

WHAT YOU NEED
- Nylon/boar-bristle brush
- Hairspray
- Hair tie

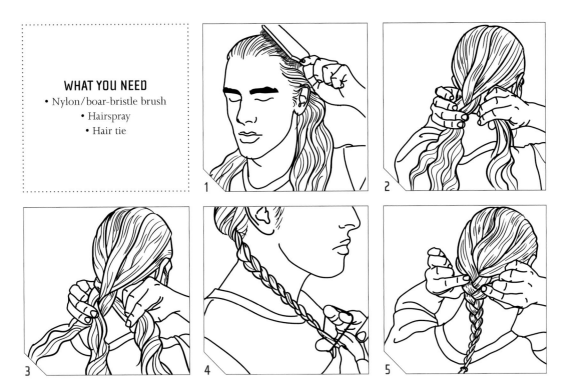

1. Start by brushing out your hair thoroughly. Make sure you get rid of any knots. When done, apply a bit of hairspray all over.

2. Now divide your hair into three equal-sized sections. Begin to braid by taking the strand that is on the right-hand side over into the middle to become the new central strand.

3. Now repeat the same thing with the section on the left-hand side, taking it over and into the middle.

4. Continue down in this way, working one outside strand and then the other until all your hair has been braided, then secure the end with a hair tie.

5. Finish off by pulling out the edges down your braid. This will prevent it from looking too neat and tight, and will give it a looser, more masculine appearance.

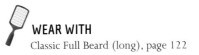

WEAR WITH
Classic Full Beard (long), page 122

BRAID INTO TOPKNOT

This style is definitely only for those who can handle a challenge! It requires you to master a new technique—the Dutch braid. This is something that you'll need to practice, but once you've learned how to do a standard three-strand braid (see page 84), then a Dutch braid is just one step beyond that, and the more complex effect is really worth the effort.

DIFFICULTY - Difficult

IDEAL FACE SHAPE - All face shapes

IDEAL HAIR - All textures, but the braid will be more visible on straight hair

WHAT YOU NEED
- Comb
- 2 hair ties

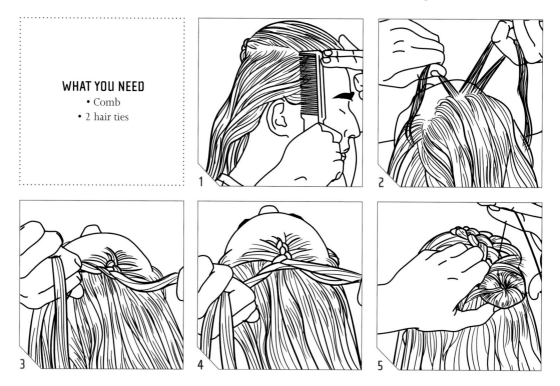

1. Separate out a top section of hair with your comb, as for the Double Bun, page 112. Tie the lower part of your hair out of the way.

2. Divide the top section into three equal strands.

3. As for a regular braid, take one outer strand into the middle, then repeat with the other outer strand. But here, each strand should pass under and up into the center to create a raised braid.

4. For the next round, incorporate a small portion of hair from one side of your head into the outer strand

on that side before taking it under and up. Do the same with the outer strand on the other side. Then continue working back in this way. Work slowly and carefully.

5. When you reach the end of the parted section, the hard bit is over! Stop braiding, twirl the remaining hair into a tight knot, and secure it with a hair tie. Release the bottom section of hair.

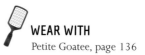

WEAR WITH
Petite Goatee, page 136

TOP TIP

Try a French braid (the reverse of a Dutch braid)—where outer strands pass over (not under) and into the center.

TOP TIP

Any brush will do for this, but you may find a detangling brush is useful if your hair is prone to knots.

HALF-UP BUN

This is a great style that's easy to throw up at a moment's notice. To start with, you might not get it looking as clean and perfect as you would like, but that's just a matter of practice. This is actually a very easy look—in my opinion, if a guy can't pull this one off, then he may as well cut off his hair!

DIFFICULTY - Easy

IDEAL FACE SHAPE - Smaller, more compact face shapes—oval or square

IDEAL HAIR - Any texture

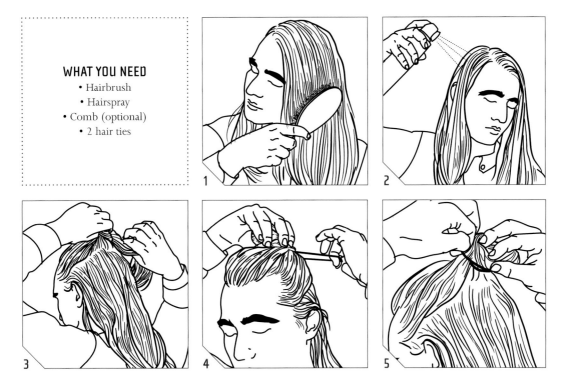

WHAT YOU NEED
- Hairbrush
- Hairspray
- Comb (optional)
- 2 hair ties

1. Start by brushing your hair thoroughly to get rid of any knots.

2. For hold, apply a light amount of hairspray all over, holding the can around 8 inches (20 cm) away from your head.

3. Now scoop the top half of your hair into a ponytail. Use a comb if you want a really neat part. Then, holding the base of the ponytail with one hand, smooth the sides and top with your brush.

4. Secure the pony with a hair tie, then take the pony with both hands and twist it at the same time as curling it up into a bun that sits on your crown. It may take a few goes to get this right.

5. Secure the bun with a second hair tie, making sure that all the hair is held in position.

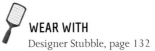

WEAR WITH
Designer Stubble, page 132

MID-PONY

If there is a classic ponytail, then this is it—hair swept back, with the base of the ponytail sitting midway up the back of the head. The chances are that if you have long hair, this is a style you've worn before. However, since it is such a simple look, it's worth taking the time to get a really clean, striking, and long-lasting result.

DIFFICULTY - Medium

IDEAL FACE SHAPE - All face shapes

IDEAL HAIR - Any texture

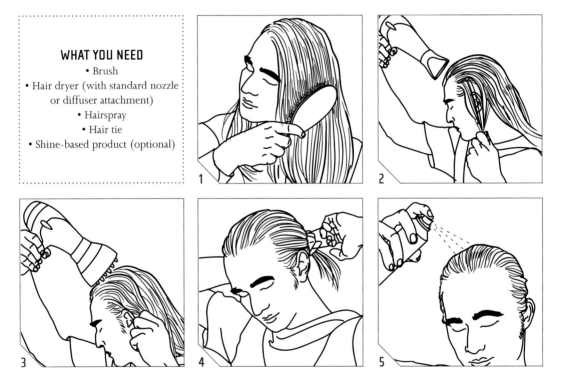

WHAT YOU NEED
- Brush
- Hair dryer (with standard nozzle or diffuser attachment)
- Hairspray
- Hair tie
- Shine-based product (optional)

1. If you choose to begin with dry hair, brush it thoroughly to get rid of any knots or tangles.

2. If starting with wet hair, you will need to blow-dry it. (If you wash your hair and put it straight into a pony while wet, it will dry in that shape!) If you have frizzy hair and want it to look sleek, then blow-dry it with the hair dryer nozzle directed down the hair shaft as you pull the hair taut with your brush.

3. If you have curly or wavy hair, using a diffuser attachment instead will avoid introducing any frizz.

4. Now apply a light mist of hairspray, then sweep your hair back to the middle of your head, keeping the sides and top as smooth as you can. Secure the pony with a hair tie.

5. Finish off with another light touch of hairspray to tame any flyaways.

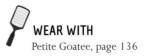

WEAR WITH
Petite Goatee, page 136

TOP TIP

For a really classy look, add some shine spray before creating the pony—or, for both shine and a bit of hold, choose a wax or pomade.

TOP TIP

Consider buying a good-quality
hairbrush for the best results.
It may cost more, but it will last
for years.

BRAIDED BUN

For this style, start with dry hair (unless you specifically want a wet look), and make sure that you apply product as recommended. Clean hair with no product on it will work against you—it will be much harder to control and manipulate, and the style will not stay in place as long.

DIFFICULTY – Medium to difficult
IDEAL FACE SHAPE – All face shapes
IDEAL HAIR – Wavy to straight

WHAT YOU NEED
- Thickening cream or salt spray
- Hair brush (ideally a nylon/boar-bristle brush)
- 2 large hair ties and 1 small hair tie

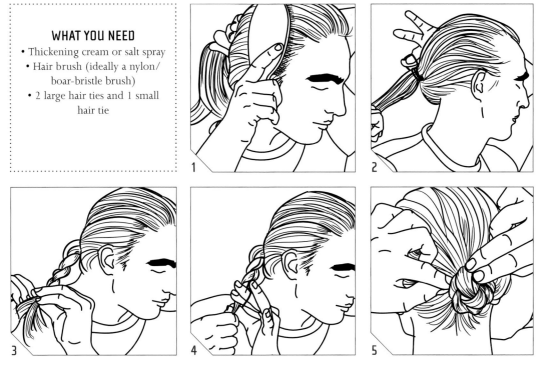

1. Brush your hair back neatly into a low ponytail, holding it in place with your free hand.

2. Secure the ponytail with one of your large hair ties.

3. Now divide your pony into three equal strands to create a three-strand braid, taking the outside strand on one side over to the middle, followed by the strand on the opposite side, and so on. (See page 84 for additional instructions if you need them.)

4. Secure the end of the braid with your small hair tie.

This will be less bulky and more secure for the small end portion of hair here.

5. Finish by coiling the braid up and around, securing it in place with your second large hair tie.

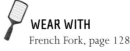

WEAR WITH
French Fork, page 128

SAMURAI PONY

This subtle but striking play on a standard pony depends on the contrast of sleek, smooth hair on the head, with the textured appearance of the ponytail at the back. Don't be afraid to use a lot of hairspray. If you find that you want more grip when creating the ponytail, just add more spray. (See also the Samurai Bun on page 102.)

DIFFICULTY – Easy

IDEAL FACE SHAPE – All face shapes

IDEAL HAIR – The longer and straighter the better!

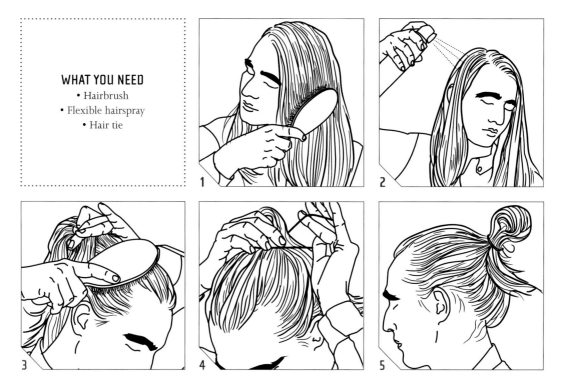

WHAT YOU NEED
• Hairbrush
• Flexible hairspray
• Hair tie

1. Start by brushing your hair really thoroughly to get rid of any knots. Work all the way round your head.

2. For hold, apply a light amount of hairspray all over, holding the can around 8 inches (20 cm) away from your head.

3. Now scoop all of your hair up into a ponytail at the crown, brushing it up from the roots as you hold it in place at the base with your other hand.

4. Secure your ponytail with a hair tie.

5. Now pull a portion of your ponytail through the hair tie, but not all the way, to create a bun shape on top, while leaving the ends hanging free below for the samurai effect.

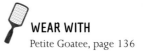

WEAR WITH
Petite Goatee, page 136

TOP TIP

Firm-hold hairspray can make hair sticky and hard to brush. Flexible spray allows you to keep brushing and layering on spray.

TOP TIP

On my model here I also used a bit of dry shampoo at the roots before starting, just for a bit of extra body.

TEXTURED LAYERS

The main thing to focus on here is building up the texture, especially at the start. Once you've applied your thickening product—be that mousse, salt spray, or spray gel—blow-dry it in, and then reapply. Keep working in this way, drying and adding, building up the product in subtle layers. Work intuitively and judge by the results—keep layering up until you have the effect you're after.

DIFFICULTY - Medium

IDEAL FACE SHAPE - All face shapes

IDEAL HAIR - Straight to wavy hair

WHAT YOU NEED
- Salt spray
- Hair dryer
- Fiber paste
- Hairspray
- Dry shampoo (optional)

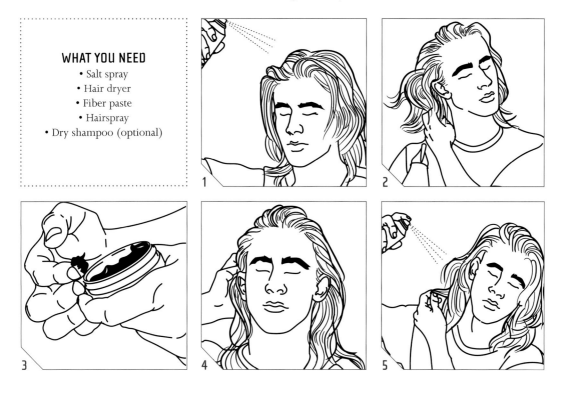

1. Start by spraying your wet hair with some salt spray.

2. Now blow-dry your hair, adding as much movement into it with your hands as you can. At this point, judge how much texture is present in the hair. Add a bit more spray then dry again. Repeat this process until you're satisfied with the texture and volume.

3. Now grab a small portion of fiber paste and warm it up between your fingers.

4. Run the paste through your hair for a final touch of messiness, then tuck your hair back behind your ears.

5. Lock it all in place with hairspray and you'll then be able to forget about it for the rest of the day.

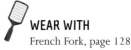

WEAR WITH
French Fork, page 128

WARRIOR BRAIDS

This style consists of a couple of three-strand braids, sitting to one side of your face, with the rest of your hair left loose. This can be a bit fiddly when you're new to it, but because the braids are created right next to your face, you can watch what you are doing in the mirror.
I created two braids here, but you could create just one.

DIFFICULTY - Medium to difficult

IDEAL FACE SHAPE - All face shapes

IDEAL HAIR - All types, but straight hair gives the most striking results

WHAT YOU NEED
- Hair brush
- Fine-tooth comb
- 2 thin elastic hair ties

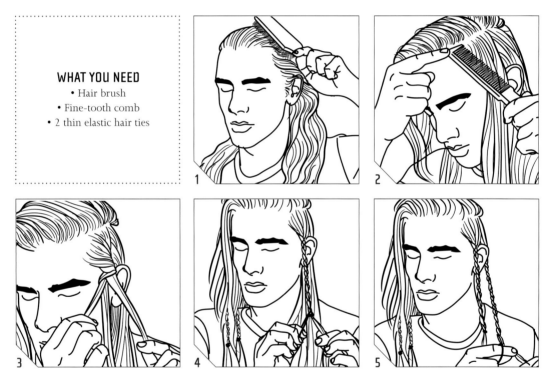

1. Begin by brushing your hair thoroughly.

2. Now separate out a small section of hair by your temple with your comb.

3. Divide the section into three equal strands, then take the strand closest to your face over the middle strand so that it becomes the new central strand. Then do the same with the strand on the far side to complete the first round of braiding. (Refer to page 84 if you need extra guidance.)

4. Continue braiding until you reach the ends and then secure the braid with a hair tie.

5. Now create a second braid in exactly the same way, just behind the first one.

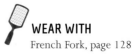

WEAR WITH
French Fork, page 128

TOP TIP

Because these braids are so subtle and thin, you'll need to use small, thin elastics. Regular hair ties will be too chunky, and will slip off the braids.

TOP TIP

If your ponytail is too tightly gathered at the nape and you want a softer effect, simply wiggle the hair above your hair tie with your fingers to loosen it.

LOW PONY

This is an incredibly straightforward style that won't take you long to master, but that doesn't mean that you can't wear it on more formal occasions—it all depends on the effort you put in. You might want to whip your hair back quickly and casually, or you may want to take the time to wash and blow-dry it before you begin for an extra-sleek finish.

DIFFICULTY - Medium

IDEAL FACE SHAPE - All face shapes

IDEAL HAIR - Any texture

WHAT YOU NEED
- Brush
- Hair dryer
(with standard nozzle or diffuser attachment)
- Hairspray
- Hair tie

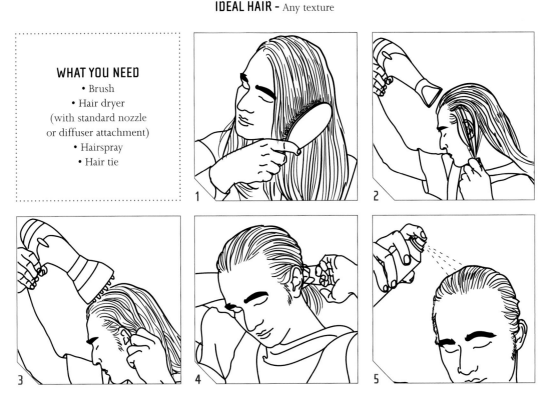

1. If you choose to begin with dry hair, brush it thoroughly to get rid of any knots or tangles.

2. If starting with wet hair, you will need to blow-dry it first, so that the hair tie doesn't create a dent in your hair! If you have frizzy hair, then direct the nozzle of your hair dryer down the hair shaft as your pull the hair taut with your brush.

3. If you have straight hair, use a diffuser instead to avoid introducing frizz.

4. Now apply a light mist of hairspray, then sweep your hair back to the nape of your neck, making sure the sides and top are kept nice and smooth. Secure the pony with a hair tie.

5. Finish off with another light touch of hairspray to tame any flyaways.

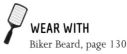

WEAR WITH
Biker Beard, page 130

SAMURAI BUN

I've called this a Samurai Bun because of the spiky hair ends sticking out of the top. This gives a nice Japanese twist to what is otherwise a very simple style. You may also want to check out the Samurai Pony on page 94 for a variation on this idea.

DIFFICULTY - Medium

IDEAL FACE SHAPE - All face shapes

IDEAL HAIR - Wavy to straight hair. Curly hair won't give you a clean finish

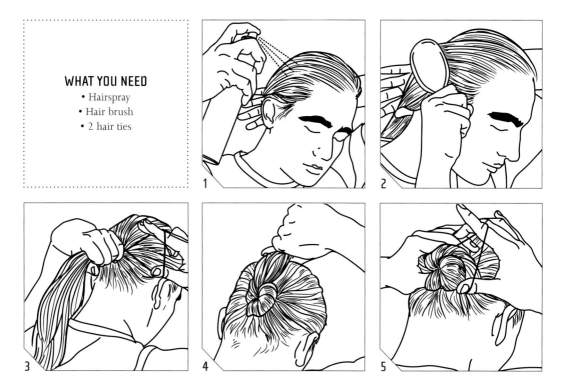

WHAT YOU NEED
- Hairspray
- Hair brush
- 2 hair ties

1. Start by giving your hair a light application of hairspray.

2. Then brush your hair into a ponytail at the back of your head. Make sure that it is brushed thoroughly and smoothly so that you end up with a very clean finish. Take your time with this.

3. When you're satisfied that the sides and top are as smooth as you can get them, secure the ponytail with a hair tie.

4. Now gently twist your ponytail around and up into a coiled bun shape.

5. Secure the bun in place with your second hair tie, making sure that the ends stick up free at the top of the bun, as shown on my model opposite.

WEAR WITH
Petite Goatee, page 136

TOP TIP

Make sure that the ends that are left free are short enough to stick straight up. You want this to look spiky and sharp, not droopy.

TOP TIP

Salt spray and hairspray may seem a lot for such a simple style, but skip these and I guarantee you will notice the difference.

TOPKNOT

The topknot is a very adaptable style, and you'll notice that there are a few in this book alone. The version I've created here is the simplest of these—a loosely created knot high on the head, with plenty of texture in the hair for a casual, unfussy effect.

DIFFICULTY – Medium

IDEAL FACE SHAPE – All face shapes

IDEAL HAIR – All textures

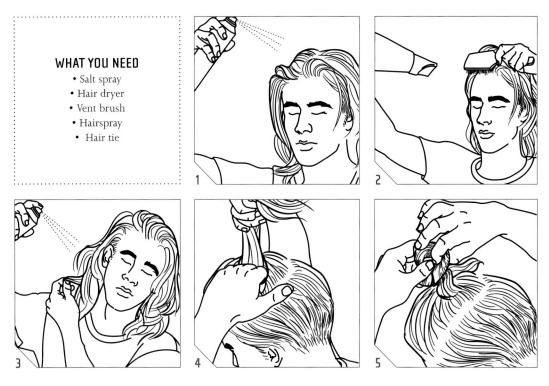

WHAT YOU NEED
- Salt spray
- Hair dryer
- Vent brush
- Hairspray
- Hair tie

1. Start with wet hair and begin by spritzing it all over with some salt spray.

2. Now dry it thoroughly using your hair dryer and a vent brush.

3. Once your hair is thoroughly dry, give it a light application of hairspray.

4. Now separate out a section of hair on top of your head—roughly about one third of your hair.

5. Take this top section up into a ponytail, and secure it with a hair tie. However, on the last twist of the tie, pull your ponytail through, but not all the way, to create the topknot shape shown opposite.

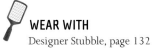

WEAR WITH
Designer Stubble, page 132

HALF-UP BRAIDED PONY

By this stage of the book, you should know how to create a simple three-strand braid. And you've already learned how to create a half-up bun. So the next obvious step is to bring the two together! Admittedly, you will be creating the braid at the back of your head, but I didn't want to make this too easy for you...

DIFFICULTY - Medium

IDEAL FACE SHAPE - All face shapes

IDEAL HAIR - Any hair type

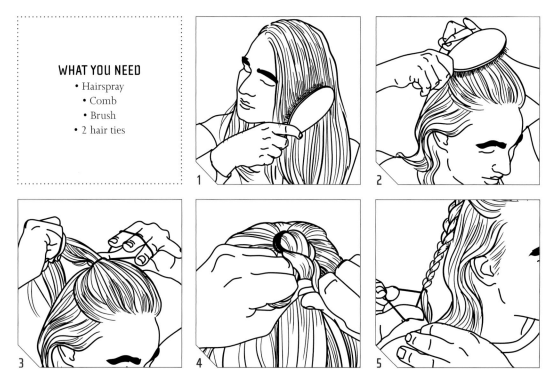

WHAT YOU NEED
- Hairspray
- Comb
- Brush
- 2 hair ties

1. Start with dry hair. Brush it out to make sure it's free of any knots and tangles, then apply a mist of hairspray all over.

2. Now separate out a section at the top of your head with a comb, then brush this top section back into a ponytail, held in place with your other hand.

3. Secure the pony with a hair tie.

4. Divide your pony into three equal strands to create a three-strand braid, taking the outside strand on one side over to the middle, followed by the strand on the opposite side, and so on. (See page 84 for additional instructions if you need them.)

5. When you reach the end, secure the ponytail with a second hair tie.

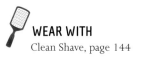

WEAR WITH
Clean Shave, page 144

TOP TIP

You may think you can skip the hairspray for this style, but don't. It will give the braid grip, and hold it in place for much longer.

TOP TIP

If your hair is not quite long
enough to create a full bun, use
some invisible pins (very thin
bobby pins that are easily
concealed) to secure any
loose ends.

EASY MAN BUN

This is one of those styles that is incredibly easy to pull off once you know how to do it—it's the sort of thing that you see women whip up in an instant without a mirror. It may seem tricky creating this on yourself to begin with, but you will get the hang of it after a few goes. It's not a style that's meant to look too perfect, anyway!

DIFFICULTY - Medium

IDEAL FACE SHAPE - All face shapes

IDEAL HAIR - Any texture

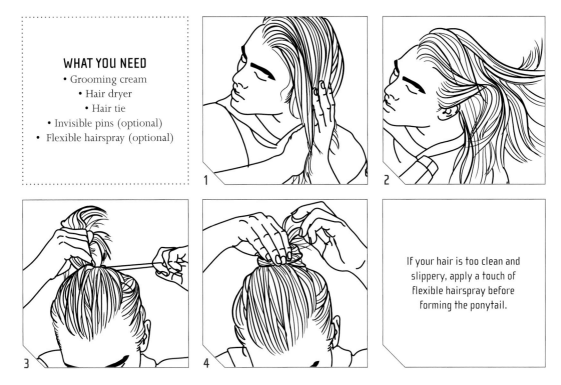

WHAT YOU NEED
- Grooming cream
- Hair dryer
- Hair tie
- Invisible pins (optional)
- Flexible hairspray (optional)

If your hair is too clean and slippery, apply a touch of flexible hairspray before forming the ponytail.

1. Start by applying some grooming cream to wet hair. This is a lightweight cream that will tame any flyaways.

2. Now blow-dry your hair. You will be putting your hair up in a bun, so you don't need to worry too much about using a brush to keep it sleek.

3. When your hair is dry, gather it all up into a ponytail at the crown of your head, then secure it with a hair tie around the base.

4. Finally, twist the ponytail around and up into a bun, arranging the hair tie so that it holds everything in place. (When you've done this a few times, you'll find that adding the tie, twisting up the bun, and securing it in place all become one fluid movement.)

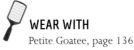

WEAR WITH
Petite Goatee, page 136

LONG AND LOOSE

This is a nice way of styling your hair if you're wanting to create some texture for a night out, but you don't want a look that is too fussy or over the top. It's very soft and simple, and yet dressy enough to complement a roll-neck sweater or a dress jacket. You do need a bit of length, but it works well on all hair textures—from straight to curly.

DIFFICULTY – Medium

IDEAL FACE SHAPE – All face shapes

IDEAL HAIR – All textures

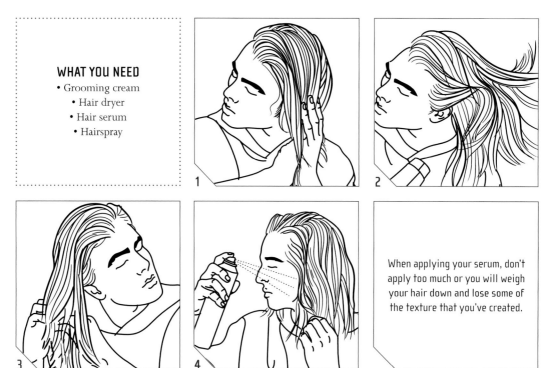

WHAT YOU NEED
- Grooming cream
- Hair dryer
- Hair serum
- Hairspray

When applying your serum, don't apply too much or you will weigh your hair down and lose some of the texture that you've created.

1. Start with wet hair. Rub a small amount of grooming cream between your fingers and then run it through the length of your hair. This will add texture and polish, and get rid of any frizz. It's a great product to use for softer styles.

2. Now give your hair a blast with the hair dryer. Keep going until your hair is completely dry. You are aiming for a textured look, so don't worry about using a brush and keeping it sleek.

3. Now apply some serum to style and finish. Warm up a very small quantity between your fingers, and then run it through your hair, distributing it evenly.

4. Finally, give your hair a touch of hairspray—just enough to keep everything in place, while also retaining the loose effect that you've created.

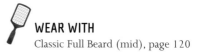

WEAR WITH
Classic Full Beard (mid), page 120

TOP TIP

Depending on what type of texture you're trying to create, you can replace the grooming cream with salt spray or a thickening spray gel.

TOP TIP

Make the triangular part as neat as you can because, once the hair is up in a bun on top, it will be highly visible. Get help with this if you need it!

DOUBLE BUN

The impact of this double bun is enhanced by the creation of a V-shaped part between the
top and bottom sections, a bit like a shark fin. Simply use a comb to part your hair on
either side, from either side of your forehead, and meeting at the back,
forming a triangular section of hair on top.

DIFFICULTY - Medium to difficult

IDEAL FACE SHAPE - All face shapes, but not square

IDEAL HAIR - Long and straight is perfect

WHAT YOU NEED
- Wide-tooth comb
- Crocodile clip
- Brush
- 4 hair ties

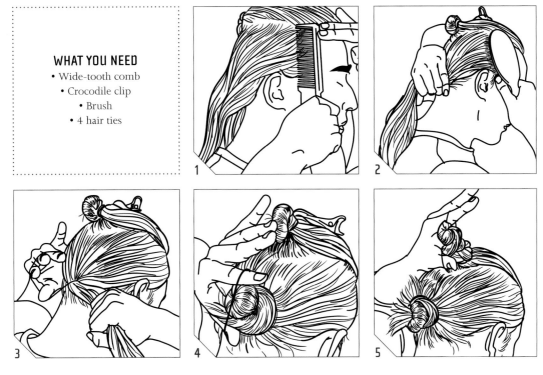

1. As mentioned above, you will need to start by
dividing your hair into an upper and lower section by
creating a V-shaped part. Clip this top section up out of
the way for now.

2. Brush the bottom half of your hair into a ponytail.
This should sit right on the occipital bone, which is at
the base of your head at the back, so that there is a
good distance between the two buns.

3. Secure the bottom ponytail with a hair tie.

4. Now coild the bottom ponytail up into a bun,
securing it with a second hair tie. (Refer to page 114
for how to do this.)

5. Now release the top section and repeat Steps 2 to 4
to create a second coiled bun on top.

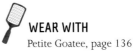

WEAR WITH
Petite Goatee, page 136

TWIST-IN BUN

Things that look casual can sometimes be trickier to master than you think, so don't skip the hairspray before you start—not only will it keep flyaways in check, it will also add hold and texture, making your hair much easier to work with. Keep the sides nice and clean, too. The focus here should be on the coil at the back of your head.

DIFFICULTY - Medium to difficult

IDEAL FACE SHAPE - All face shapes

IDEAL HAIR - Medium to thick; trickier with finer hair

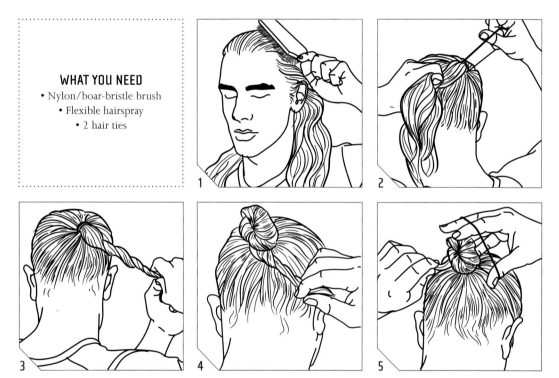

WHAT YOU NEED
- Nylon/boar-bristle brush
- Flexible hairspray
- 2 hair ties

1. Start by brushing your dry hair thoroughly and then applying plenty of flexible hairspray—this will give your hair hold without it becoming too stiff and unworkable. You can also create this style with wet hair, but it will be slippery to work with.

2. Now create a ponytail at the back of your head and secure it with a hair tie.

3. Next, twist the ponytail, holding the end secure.

4. Now, keeping hold of the twist that you've created, coil it up into a bun, circling it firmly around the hair tie. Coil the ends right round and tuck them neatly under the bun.

5. Finish by securing the bun with your second hair tie, tucking any last stray hairs into place.

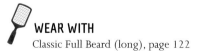 **WEAR WITH**
Classic Full Beard (long), page 122

TOP TIP

Make sure to secure the end of your pony with the second tie or the twist will unravel!

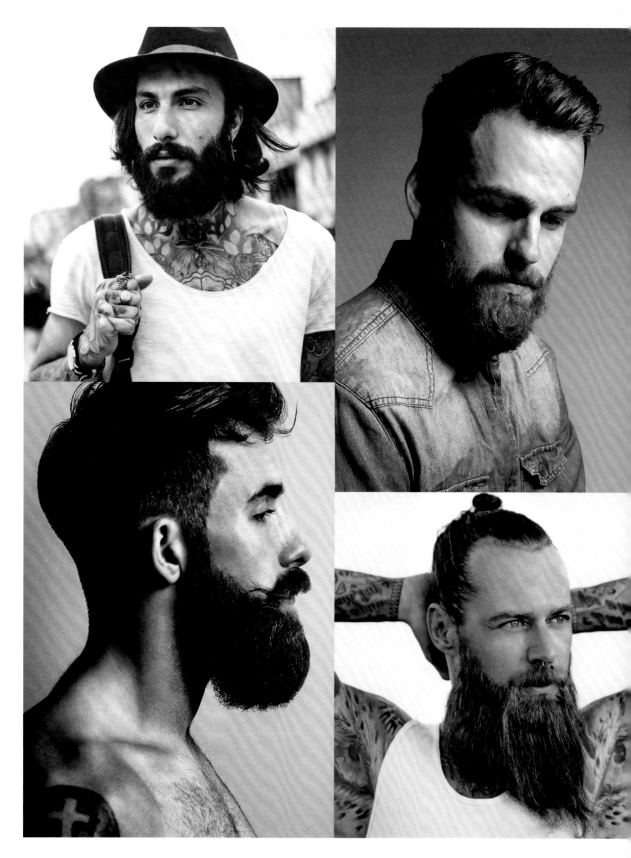

CHAPTER 4

CLASSIC FULL BEARD (SHORT)

Although the classic full beard is a look worn by many, there are all sorts of lengths out there. For simplicity I have focused on three key lengths in this chapter—short, mid, and long. For the short option, the key to good-looking results is keeping the beard even and tight to the face. Make sure that you create nice clean edges for a really defined look.

DIFFICULTY - Easy

IDEAL FACE SHAPE - All face shapes

WHAT YOU NEED
- Beard trimmer
- Beard balm

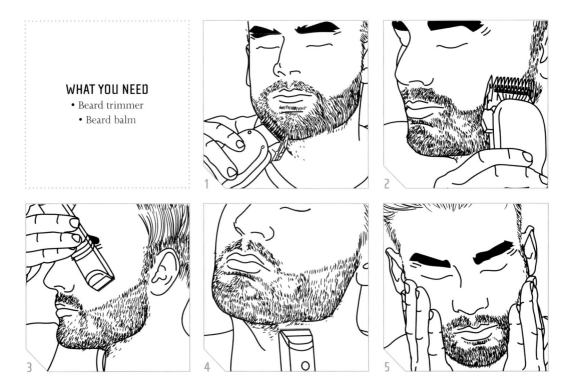

1. Start by using your trimmer to trim your beard down. Here, I used a no. 2 guard for a 6-mm trim all over. Start at one side of the beard.

2. Now move to the sideburn area and trim this back to the same length.

3. Next, use your trimmer without a guard to create the line on the top, curving into the sideburn area.

4. Then do the same under your chin.

5. Finally apply a bit of beard balm to your facial hair with your fingers, working in the direction of growth. This will condition the hair and keep it looking neat.

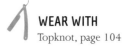

WEAR WITH
Topknot, page 104

TOP TIP

Beard balm is part moisturizer, part sealant. It helps with styling, but also keeps your beard looking healthy and full.

TOP TIP

You may find it easier to finish off
the hair around your lips with a
pair of grooming scissors.

CLASSIC FULL BEARD (MID)

The idea here is to create something halfway in between the short and long versions of a classic full beard, but you also want to concentrate on achieving a slightly rounder shape with this one. This is can be useful for softening an overly square or angular face.

DIFFICULTY – Easy

IDEAL FACE SHAPE – All face shapes

WHAT YOU NEED
- Comb
- Beard trimmer
- Beard balm or oil

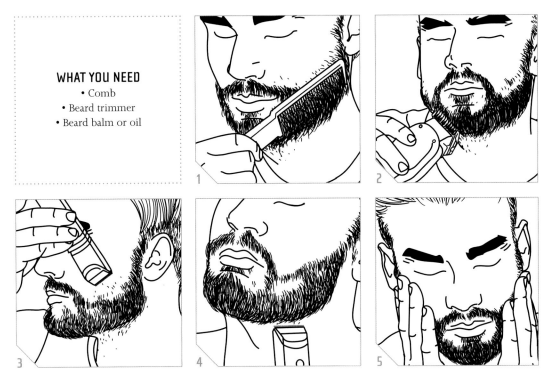

1. Start by combing through your beard so that all the hairs are fully extended and will not get missed by the trimmer.

2. Now attach your chosen guard to your trimmer and begin to take back the length around the chin. Follow around to either side, making sure you maintain a consistent length overall.

3. Now remove the guard and create a nice clean line above the beard, lining your cheeks.

4. Then do the same under your chin.

5. Finally, warm up a bit of beard balm or oil between your palms, then work it through your beard, sweeping the hair in the direction of growth.

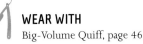

WEAR WITH
Big-Volume Quiff, page 46

CLASSIC FULL BEARD (LONG)

The trick here is to avoid creating just a messy, bushy beard. Instead, focus on forming a decisive, triangular shape by trimming neatly around the edges of the beard, and angling it down toward the tip. Keep combing as you work so that you spot any stray bits and pieces. Although this is a full beard, you want it to look groomed and deliberate.

DIFFICULTY - Medium

IDEAL FACE SHAPE - All face shapes

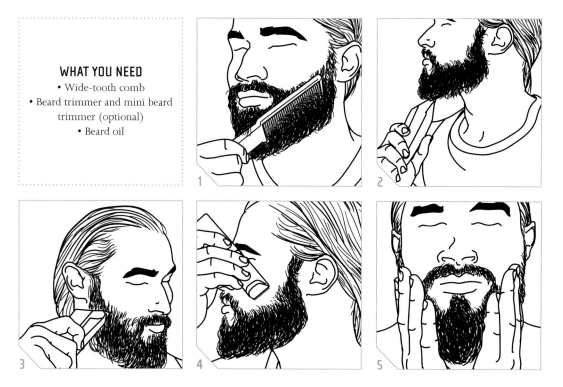

WHAT YOU NEED
- Wide-tooth comb
- Beard trimmer and mini beard trimmer (optional)
- Beard oil

1. Start by brushing out your beard with a comb so that all the hairs are fully extended.

2. Now start to shape your beard with your trimmer, using the guard that matches your desired length. Start at the front and work to the back (the neck).

3. Next, reduce a bit of bulk and refine the shape, working down from the side to the front. Do the same thing on both sides.

4. Now tidy up the edges of your beard with a smaller clipper, or change the guard to get a closer shave. Create a nice line to define the cheekbones.

5. Finish by warming a few drops of beard oil in your palms and then smoothing it through your beard.

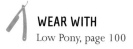

WEAR WITH
Low Pony, page 100

TOP TIP

Beard oil will not only moisturize your beard, but will also give it a healthy-looking sheen.

TOP TIP

Always work from long to short.
Trim to 13mm first, then start to
taper back from that.

TAPERED BEARD

As the name suggests, the all-important thing here is to achieve a shape that tapers gradually from the longest point at your chin, back to shortest point right up by the top of your ear. Make sure you comb out your beard both before and after to check that the taper is exactly the way you want it.

DIFFICULTY – Medium

IDEAL FACE SHAPE – All face shapes

WHAT YOU NEED
- Comb
- Beard trimmer
- Beard balm

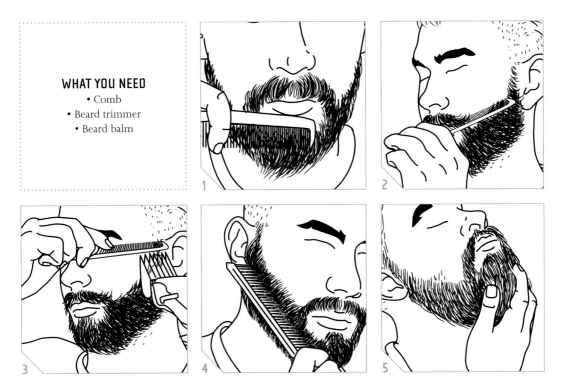

1. Start by combing out your beard so that you can see its current shape clearly.

2. Now use your comb to determine where the taper should start and finish by combing the hair in an upward direction.

3. Open the taper arm or lever on your trimmer (the longest setting) and attach a no. 4 (13mm) guard for the longest areas, then graduate down to a no. 2 (6mm) guard where you want to taper in tighter. Work

from mid-ear up to the top of the ear, flicking out the clipper in a C-shaped motion at the top to blend.

4. When complete, comb the sides down to check that the shape is as you intended.

5. Finally, work some balm through the beard.

 WEAR WITH
Slickback, page 52

SQUARE BEARD

A well-defined, heavy, square beard can give you a striking, contemporary look. You'll be working both with and without a guard, so you need to make sure that you work with a steady hand. Remember, too, to keep checking the shape as you work, so that you maintain the correct outline.

DIFFICULTY - Medium

IDEAL FACE SHAPE - All face shapes, but not overly broad faces

WHAT YOU NEED
- Comb
- Beard trimmer
- Beard balm

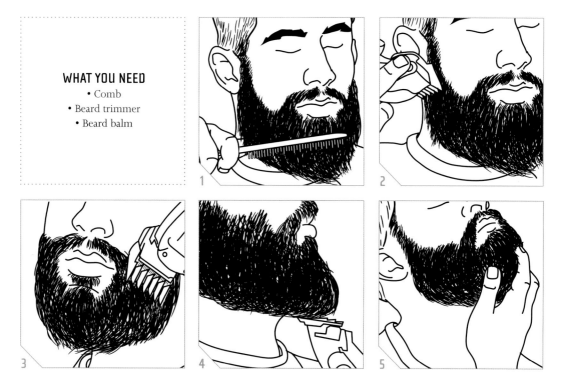

1. Begin by combing out your beard thoroughly in preparation for trimming.

2. Start on one side, by the top of the ear, using your beard trimmer with a no. 1 or 2 (4.5–6mm) guard attached. Work in a downward motion to create a square shape. Although you are using a guard here, you need to make sure that the shape stays square, rather than simply following the outline of your face. Repeat this on the other side.

3. Continue down to and around the chin on both sides, preserving the correct shape.

4. Now remove the guard and work freehand to create the square shape under your chin.

5. Finally, warm up a bit of beard balm in your fingers, then run it through to tame and shape your beard.

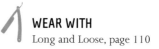

WEAR WITH
Long and Loose, page 110

TOP TIP

Keep the shape under the chin blocky and straight to emphasize the overall effect.

TOP TIP

Work slowly, making sure that the beard tapers symmetrically, from short to long on both sides, or the impact of the fork will be weaker.

FRENCH FORK

The name of this style comes from its distinctive forked front. To give yourself the right starting point for creating this, you need to ensure that you maintain enough length in the chin area. The beard should be shortest at the jaw, graduating out to its fullest right where the fork will sit.

DIFFICULTY - Medium

IDEAL FACE SHAPE - All face shapes; can helpfully elongate a round face

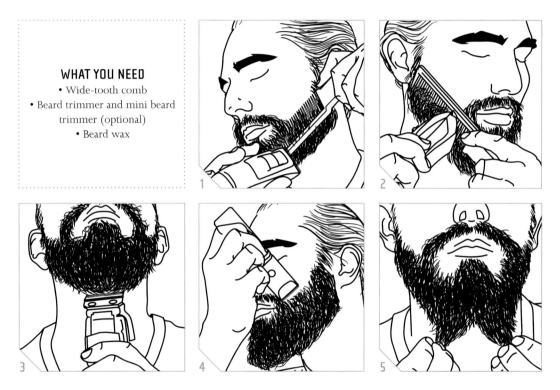

WHAT YOU NEED
• Wide-tooth comb
• Beard trimmer and mini beard trimmer (optional)
• Beard wax

1. Hold your comb down one side of your beard, at a distance that matches your desired length, with any excess hair sticking through the teeth of the comb. Trim this hair away. Grade the shape, keeping it long at the front, and shorter at the jaw.

2. Repeat this on the other side.

3. Lift your chin up and trim the underside of the beard, but don't lose any of the length here.

4. Tidy the edges on your jaw and cheeks with a mini trimmer, or by changing your trimmer guard for a closer shave.

5. Now warm some wax in your fingers, grab the front of your beard in two equal halves, and twist them together to create your fork shape.

WEAR WITH
Low Pony, page 100

BIKER BEARD

This is a timeless look, but it does depend on having strong features. I also think it only really works on oval or triangular face shapes—I'd avoid this one if you have a very square jawline, or a very rounded face, because you will struggle to get the right effect. Make sure the rest of your face is quite clean-shaven so that the beard remains the dominant element.

DIFFICULTY - Easy

IDEAL FACE SHAPE - Oval or triangular faces are best

WHAT YOU NEED
- Beard trimmer
- Grooming scissors
- Beard balm or wax

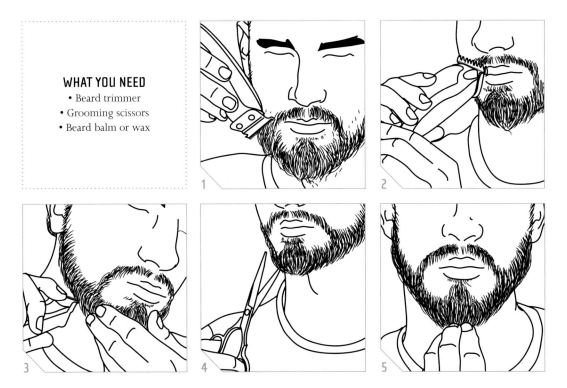

1. Start by "lining" your beard, edging in to create the desired shape. Do this on both sides.

2. Now move on to your mustache, if you have one. Either remove this, or trim it very close to the face. The focus should be very much on the beard.

3. Next, move on to cleaning up the sides with your trimmer.

4. Then trim off any excess hair from the beard using your scissors to get the desired shape.

5. Finally, apply some beard balm or beard wax. Wax will help define and hold the shape and make it stand out from the face a bit more, if that is your preference. Use your fingertips to perfect the look.

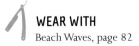

WEAR WITH
Beach Waves, page 82

TOP TIP

Talking and eating can dislodge a neat mustache, so use wax if you want to avoid this!

TOP TIP

Don't switch hands when you
switch to the second side—use
your dominant hand for both
sides of your face.

DESIGNER STUBBLE

Stubble can simply look like two-day growth! If you want a much more preened look, the trick is to keep the edges nice and clean for definition. You'll know your own face shape best, and with practice you'll get used to shaping this in a way that expresses your personality. What length you go for is your choice: this look is all about the shape.

DIFFICULTY – Easy

IDEAL FACE SHAPE – All face shapes

WHAT YOU NEED
- Beard trimmer
- Cut-throat razor
- Aftershave balm or cooling moisturizer
- Towel and water

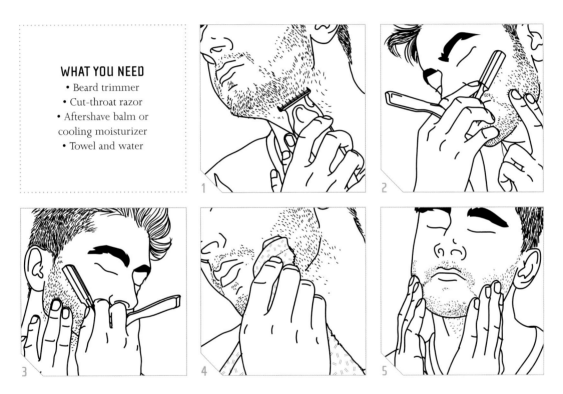

1. Start by taking your beard down with your trimmer, pulling your skin taut to reduce razor burn.

2. Next, use your cut-throat razor to "line" the beard to the desired shape. Hold the razor at a 30-degree angle, and use small strokes to create a visually strong line. Hold your razor firmly, but don't press it into the face. Remember—a cut-throat razor is very sharp. If you don't have a cut-throat razor, you can use a regular razor, although the results will not be as precise.

3. Now shave the other side of your face in the same way.

4. Wash your face to remove any loose hairs, then pat it dry with a towel. Don't rub your face—vigorous movements will cause irritation.

5. Finish off by applying some balm or moisturizer to calm your skin, soothe any razor burn, and keep your skin soft.

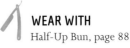

WEAR WITH
Half-Up Bun, page 88

FULL GOATEE

This is a classic, timeless style that can be worn by any man who wants to look...well, manly! A goatee restricts all facial hair to the upper lip, chin, and jaw, and this full version has the 'tache connected to the beard. (See the Petite Goatee on page 136 for a goatee with a break in it.)

DIFFICULTY - Medium

IDEAL FACE SHAPE - All shapes

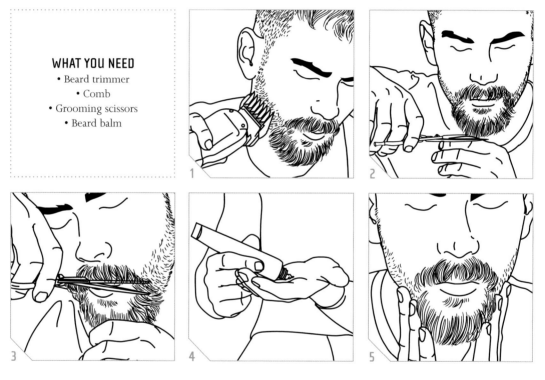

WHAT YOU NEED
- Beard trimmer
- Comb
- Grooming scissors
- Beard balm

1. Start by trimming down the sides around your beard, selecting the guard you want based on the desired length. There should be a nice strong contrast between the goatee and the rest of your facial hair.

2. Now comb the hair of your beard straight, then trim any stray, protruding hairs around the center of the goat with your scissors.

3. Do the same with your mustache, taking care to create a neat, symmetrical finish.

4. Now warm a small drop of beard balm between your palms.

5. Apply the liquefied balm to your goatee to finish, sweeping the hair in the desired direction.

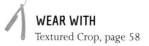

WEAR WITH
Textured Crop, page 58

TOP TIP

Don't skip the balm—it will condition the hair and keep strays in place, especially if your beard is dense, as with my model here.

TOP TIP

Retain a minimum length of around ⅜ inch (10mm) or the goatee won't stand out enough.

PETITE GOATEE

A goatee can be connected, or it may feature a break between beard and 'tache, as I've gone for here. As with the Full Goatee on page 134, this is a matter of shaving everywhere else, and leaving a thick, bushy area of hair, but here it is reduced to a much smaller area. Watch out for length, too—if you want it to stand out, make sure that you don't take it too low.

DIFFICULTY - Easy

IDEAL FACE SHAPE - All face shapes

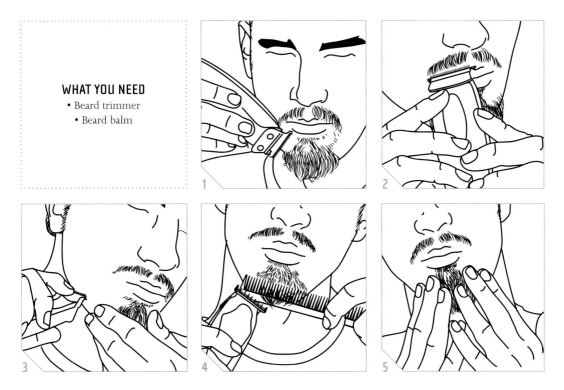

WHAT YOU NEED
- Beard trimmer
- Beard balm

1. Begin by "lining" your beard—edging in with your trimmer to create the desired shape. Do this on both sides of your beard.

2. Now move on to your mustache and do the same.

3. Next, clean up the sides with the trimmer.

4. If you want to take everything down a bit in length, you can either use the guard on the trimmer to establish your final length, or you can use a comb to do the same job. Position the comb over the hair to your chosen depth level, and then, holding it in place as a guard, trim away the excess hair sticking through it.

5. Finally, apply some beard balm, or beard oil if you feel you need some extra conditioning.

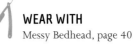

WEAR WITH
Messy Bedhead, page 40

TOP TIP

You will need a mini trimmer to be able to create the intricate lines of this style.

DEFINED LINES

Rappers are always at the forefront when it comes to hair and fashion, so it's not surprising that they've sparked off a trend in beards like the one shown here. This look is designed to make a statement, so make sure that you contrast the dense hair of the mustache and beard with very clean lines throughout.

DIFFICULTY – Medium

IDEAL FACE SHAPE – All face shapes

WHAT YOU NEED
- Mini beard trimmer

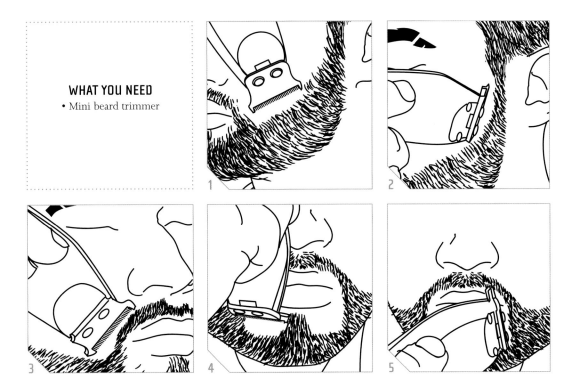

1. Start shaping your beard by creating a sharp line with your trimmer following the shape of your face, being sure to curve the line toward the top of the ear. Use the trimmer without a guard.

2. Follow on in the same way, continuing the curved shape down the side of your face on either side.

3. Next, use your trimmer to create a sharp line around your mustache. Work down the sides, and make sure your lines intersect neatly with those along your jaw.

4. Now create a boxed shape below your bottom lip using the corner of the trimmer.

5. Finally, tidy up the line between the mustache and the boxed line below the bottom lip, and clean up under the top lip.

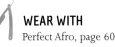

WEAR WITH
Perfect Afro, page 60

ROUNDED BEARD

Once you've perfected the Classic Full Beard you may want to start playing with shapes that do not simply follow the contours of your face, and this rounded alternative is a good place to start. You will be working freehand here, so the key thing is to take your time and make sure that you produce a result that looks deliberate.

DIFFICULTY – Medium

IDEAL FACE SHAPE – All bar very round faces!

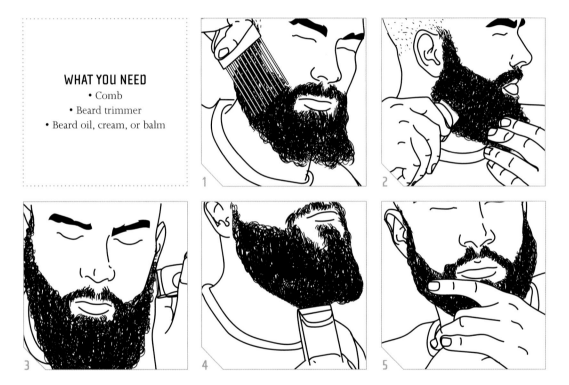

WHAT YOU NEED
- Comb
- Beard trimmer
- Beard oil, cream, or balm

1. Start by combing through your beard.

2. Now begin to create the rounded shape at the sides using your beard trimmer without a guard. You're working freehand here, so make sure the length is consistent on both sides.

3. Continue creating the round shape, and graduating the sides so that they progress from shorter at the ear to longer at the jawline.

4. Keep on working freehand, finishing off the shape around the chin.

5. Once the shape is complete, apply a beard oil, cream, or balm to tame and control the shape while also adding hydration.

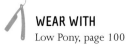

WEAR WITH
Low Pony, page 100

TOP TIP

Combing before you start will
ensure the hairs are lying flat and
extended and won't get missed by
the trimmer.

TOP TIP

This is a look that requires maintenance. Keep the areas around the mustache and beard looking clean.

MOVIE STAR

Once worn by matinee idols, this is a look that's now become synonymous with Johnny Depp. A modern "Depp" frames the face neatly, and can even make it look slimmer. The main thing, though—as with all facial-hair styles—is to make sure you keep to the contours of your own face to create a style that is individual and suits you.

DIFFICULTY - Easy

IDEAL FACE SHAPE - Oval and square are best

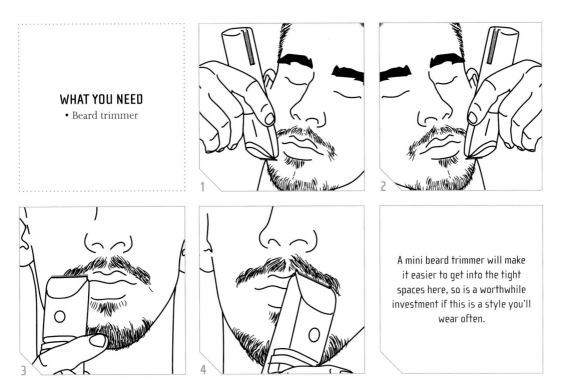

WHAT YOU NEED
• Beard trimmer

A mini beard trimmer will make it easier to get into the tight spaces here, so is a worthwhile investment if this is a style you'll wear often.

1. Start by "lining" your beard. Choose where you want the edge of your beard to be, then starting on one side of your face, apply the trimmer to your chin (with the blade pointing downward), and begin.

2. Now repeat the same thing on the other side of your face, keeping level with the shape that you created on the first side.

3. Next, line up your trimmer with the base of your mustache on one side. Again, make sure that you have decided where you want your line to be before you start trimming.

4. Now finish by completing the other side of your mustache to match. Tidy up the top of the mustache, too, if it needs it.

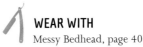

WEAR WITH
Messy Bedhead, page 40

CLEAN SHAVE

A clean shave is something you will have done many times, but it's worth taking your time to do it properly. I will talk you through how the professionals do it, taking the time to prepare the skin with a hot towel, using a brush to create a lather, and then following a 14-step process for the most thorough shave possible. You can use a disposable razor, but I recommend a safety razor for a cleaner shave.

DIFFICULTY – Easy

IDEAL FACE SHAPE – All face shapes

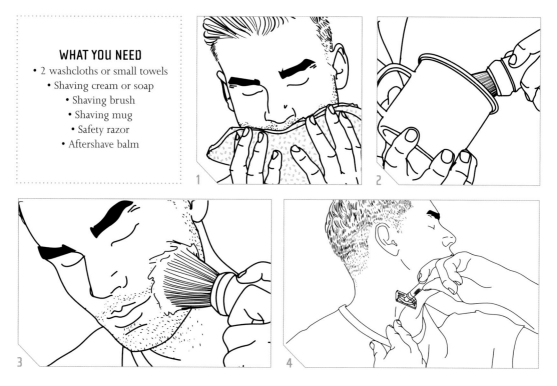

WHAT YOU NEED
- 2 washcloths or small towels
- Shaving cream or soap
- Shaving brush
- Shaving mug
- Safety razor
- Aftershave balm

1. Start by washing your face. Then prepare your hot towel by holding it under the faucet. When it is damp and steamy, wring it out, then hold it over your beard to soften the hair, making it easier to cut.

2. Put a bit of hot water in your shaving mug. Then take your brush, dampen it, and then swirl it around on your soap. Now create a thick, creamy lather by swirling your brush round in the mug. Alternatively, you can work up a lather direct on your face.

3. Apply the brush to your face with a circular motion. This movement will lift the hairs away from your face, allowing the razor to catch them all. It will also help prevent razor burn and bumps, while the warmth of the lather will further soften the hair.

4. When you begin shaving, make sure that you hold your skin taut with your free hand.

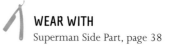

WEAR WITH
Superman Side Part, page 38

TOP TIP

When shaving, always go with the grain. Going against it will cause irritation and ingrown hairs.

TOP TIP

To prepare your cold towel, hold
a cloth under cold running water,
then wring it out.

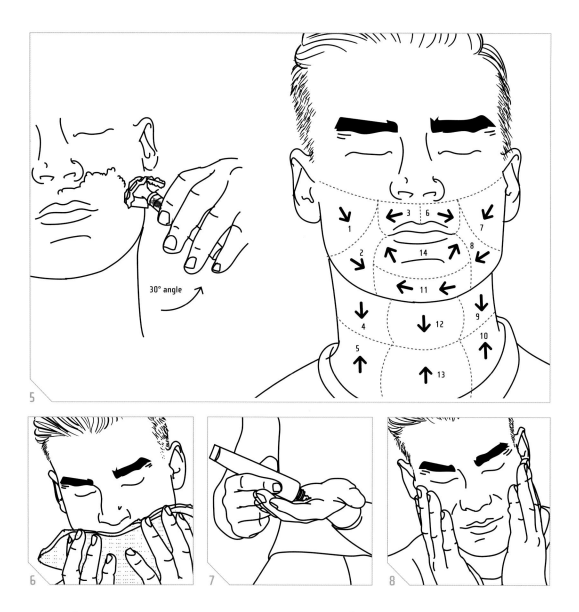

5. You will now be starting a 14-step shaving process, referring to the diagram shown here. Making sure that you go with the grain of the beard growth, start at position 1, and then follow the sequence as marked. Make sure that you always keep your razor at a 30-degree angle, too.

6. Once the shave is done, remove any excess cream with water, then apply a cold, damp towel to your face to reduce any redness or razor burn.

7. Finish off by squeezing out a bit of aftershave balm and warming it between your palms.

8. Apply the balm to your face gently to soothe the skin and moisturize it.

WEAR WITH
Superman Side Part, page 38

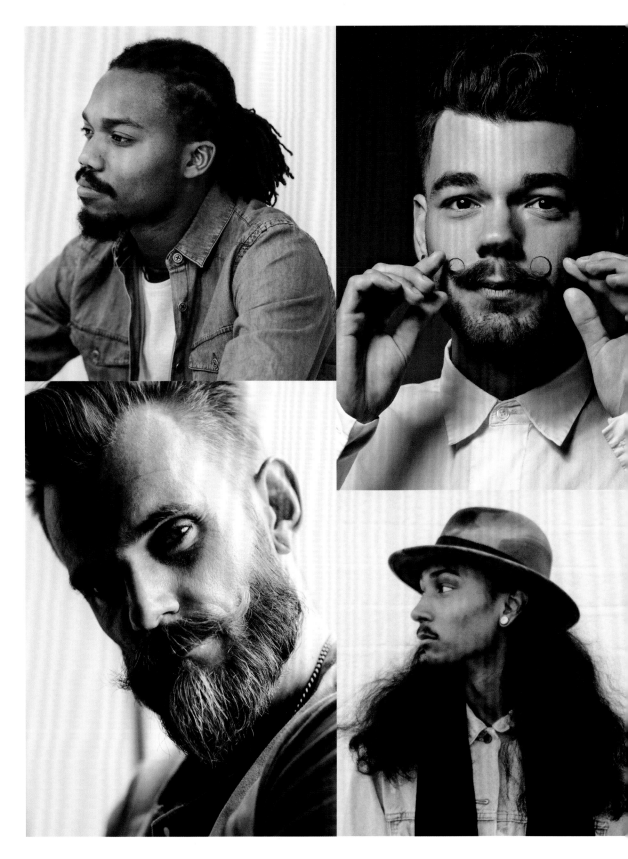

CHAPTER 5

TOP TIP

Work slowly and carefully—you
can always trim further, but it
isn't as easy to fix mistakes!

SIDEBURNS

Even if sideburns are most obvious when seen in profile, you will still want to create a symmetrical result. But there's a simple way to ensure this—you have two ears and two eyes, so use them as your guide! You can also use the straight edge of your trimmer blade to create a neat line at the base of your 'burns.

DIFFICULTY - Easy

IDEAL FACE SHAPE - All shapes

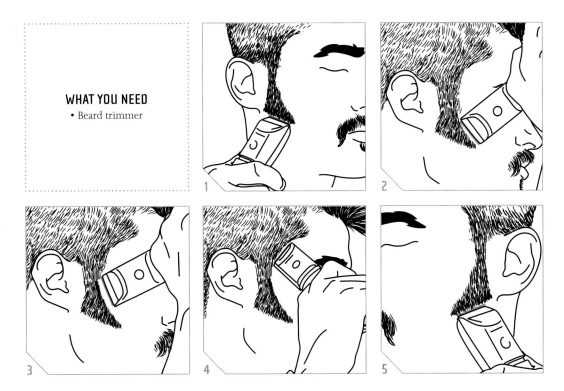

WHAT YOU NEED
• Beard trimmer

1. Start on one side, creating a nice straight line by using your trimmer to create the desired bottom line of one sideburn.

2. You will now be working in a sort of reverse circular motion to create the sideburn curve. Start at the bottom of the curve, again, positioning the trimmer to create the desired shape.

3. Continue upward, creating the right amount of curve as you go.

4. Complete the curve right up to the top, where the sideburn meets your hair at the temple.

5. Once you have the perfect shape, you are ready to repeat Steps 1 to 4 on the other side, making sure that the bottom is level on each side.

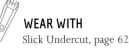

WEAR WITH
Slick Undercut, page 62

FULL 'TACHE

There is no getting round the fact that you will need plenty of hair for this style! Hair that is too sparse, or too short, just won't have the right effect. But if you have thicker, coarser hair, and the patience to let it reach the right length, then this can be a really strong look.

DIFFICULTY - Easy

IDEAL FACE SHAPE - All face shapes

WHAT YOU NEED
- Beard trimmer
- Moisturizer
- Beard balm

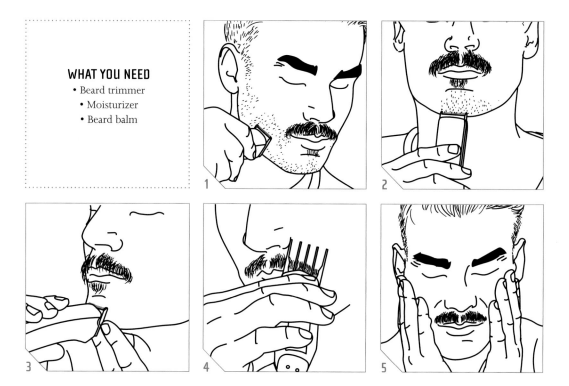

1. Start by removing the guard from your trimmer and cleaning up any stubble around the mustache. Work on the side of your jaw, right up to, but not touching, the mustache itself.

2. Do the same under your chin.

3. Make sure that you include the small area on your chin, too. The cleaner everything is, the more the focus will be on the mustache.

4. Now trim down your mustache on both sides. The standard length for a full 'tache like this is around 6 to 10 mm, so select a trimmer guard based on your preference within this range.

5. Finish by applying a bit of moisturizer to the shaved areas of your face. Use beard balm for your 'tache if you want extra sheen.

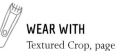

WEAR WITH
Textured Crop, page 58

TOP TIP

If you want to get rid of all signs of stubble, refer to page 144 for how to get the perfect clean shave.

TOP TIP

This is another style where investing in a mini trimmer will make the job much quicker and easier.

THIN 'TACHE

I struggled long and hard to think of a creative name for this style, but in the end I decided it was better to be clear than creative! Essentially, this is similar to the Full 'Tache (page 152), but cleaner and more streamlined. Where the full version overhangs the top lip, this sits slighty away from it, so make sure that you shave a very precise, neat line.

DIFFICULTY – Easy

IDEAL FACE SHAPE – All face shapes

WHAT YOU NEED
• Beard trimmer
• Aftershave balm or moisturizer

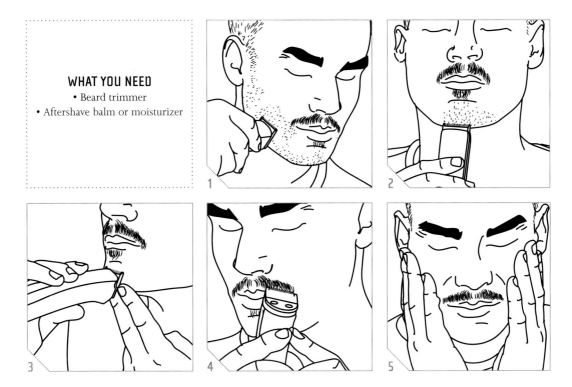

1. Start by removing the guard from your trimmer and cleaning up any stubble around the mustache. Work on the side of your jaw, right up to, but not touching, the mustache itself.

2. Do the same under the chin.

3. Make sure that you include the dent in your chin.

4. The final area to trim is the thin strip of skin between your top lip and your mustache. Use your trimmer to produce a neat line all the way along, keeping the edge parallel to your top lip.

5. Finish by applying a bit of moisturizer or balm to the shaved areas of your face.

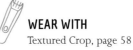

WEAR WITH
Textured Crop, page 58

CURLY 'TACHE

You do need a bit of confidence to pull off this dramatic, Salvador Dalí–inspired look, but why not test it out in the safety of your own home first? You will need sufficient length in your mustache to create the ends properly.

DIFFICULTY - Easy

IDEAL FACE SHAPE - All face shapes

WHAT YOU NEED
- Beard trimmer
- Mustache wax

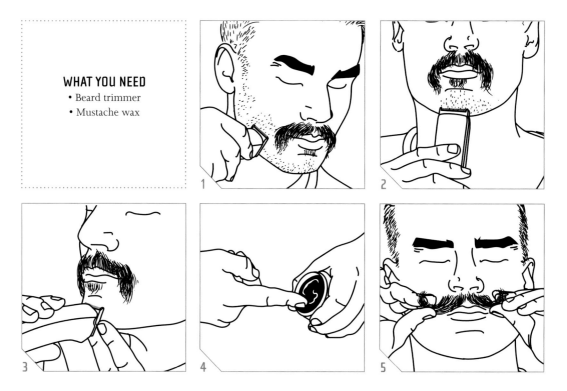

1. You can wear a curly 'tache with a beard, as shown opposite, or you can opt for a clean-shaven look everywhere else. If so, start by shaving around the mustache itself. You can either use a beard trimmer, as shown above, or you could do a wet shave (see page 144). Start by shaving the sides of your face.

2. Shave under your chin.

3. Shave the chin itself, making sure you follow all the contours of your face for a close shave.

4. Take a tiny dab of mustache wax and warm it up between your fingers.

5. Now apply the wax to the ends, twisting them up into the desired shape, as shown.

WEAR WITH
Big-Volume Quiff, page 46

TOP TIP

You won't be able to achieve this look without wax, but don't load too much on—it will weigh the ends down.

TOP TIP

Mustache wax is key here for achieving a dramatic, bold shape. Clean hair will lack hold.

HANDLEBAR 'TACHE

Creating this striking 'tache is a lot easier than you think. You need to create a distinctive shape that is slightly thinner in the center, and then widens as it extends to the sides, with downturned tips, but I'll show you a handy trick for achieving this, using your comb. As always, it's just a matter of taking your time, and practicing.

DIFFICULTY - Easy

IDEAL FACE SHAPE - Oval, square, and longer faces

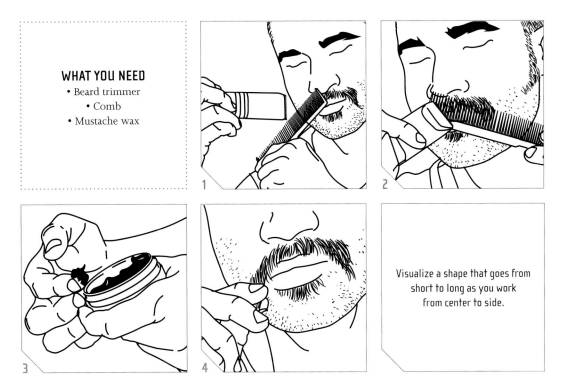

WHAT YOU NEED
- Beard trimmer
- Comb
- Mustache wax

Visualize a shape that goes from short to long as you work from center to side.

1. Place your comb over your mustache on a diagonal. This will act as your guide, so make sure that you're happy with the line before moving on. Now, holding the comb in place, use your trimmer to trim the hairs sticking through the comb, back to your chosen line and length.

2. Then do the same on the other side of your mustache, making sure that you keep the shape symmetrical.

3. Next, take a tiny bit of mustache wax and warm it up between your fingertips.

4. Finish off by applying the wax to your 'tache and tweaking the ends to get the exact shape you want.

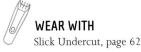

WEAR WITH
Slick Undercut, page 62

PENCIL 'TACHE

The pencil 'tache will suit anyone, but it's a unique look, so you do need the confidence to pull
it off. Although it's easy to do, one of the things that most guys get wrong when they create this is that
they cut too much off. So, as with other styles in this book, you will be using your comb as a guide,
keeping strictly to your desired line and removing exactly the right amount of excess hair.

DIFFICULTY – Easy

IDEAL FACE SHAPE – All face shapes

WHAT YOU NEED
- Beard trimmer
- Comb
- Safety razor
- Shaving gel, foam, or cream

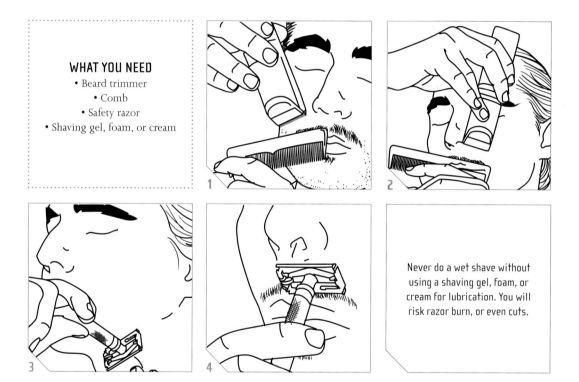

Never do a wet shave without
using a shaving gel, foam, or
cream for lubrication. You will
risk razor burn, or even cuts.

1. The key here is to use the comb and the trimmer in
tandem. Place the comb on your lip where you want
the pencil 'tache to sit and, using the comb as a guide,
remove any excess hair with the trimmer. Start on
one side.

2. Now trim the other side in the same way.

3. Finish off by shaving the sides of your face clean,
using a razor and your choice of shaving product.

4. Make sure that you work carefully around the edges
of the pencil shape.

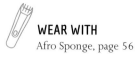

WEAR WITH
Afro Sponge, page 56

TOP TIP

I really recommend purchasing a safety razor for looks like this. You'll get good results, and also avoid nicking your skin.

TOP TIP

Keep sideburns consistent with your hair—the longer your hair, the fuller your 'burns can afford to be.

CLASSIC SIDEBURNS

Sideburns have a habit of coming in and out of fashion, in lots of shapes and lengths. Right now they're in, but if you're unsure whether they'll suit you, this subtle version is a great place to start. If you want a more stylized, retro shape, check out the variation on page 150. Whichever option you choose, though, remember that symmetry is key.

DIFFICULTY - Easy

IDEAL FACE SHAPE - All face shapes

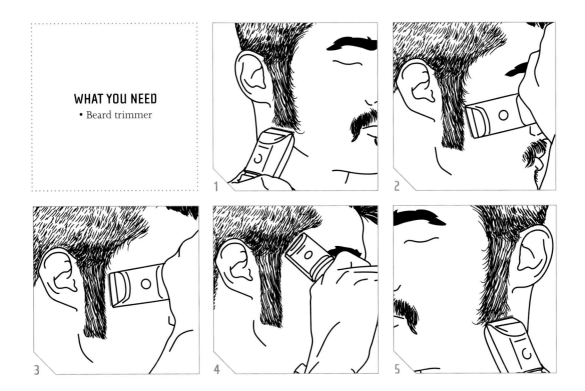

WHAT YOU NEED
• Beard trimmer

1. Starting on one side, use your trimmer without a guard to create the bottom line of one sideburn. Keep this neat and horizontal.

2. Now use your trimmer to create the line where the sideburn frames your face. Start at the bottom and work your way up. It can be good to assess your face and decide on the exact line you want, from base to temple, before you commit with the trimmer.

3. Continue up, keeping your line straight.

4. Finish at the point where the sideburns meet your hair.

5. Once you are happy with the results, repeat the same process on the other side. Take your time, checking regularly that you are creating a mirror image.

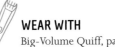

WEAR WITH
Big-Volume Quiff, page 46

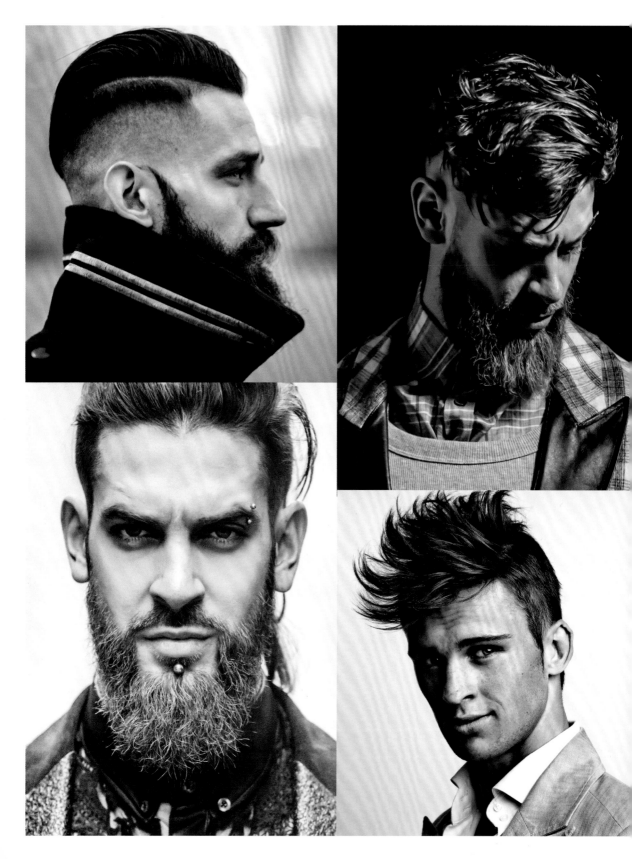

CHAPTER 6

RESOURCES

GLOSSARY

BANGS

Also referred to as a fringe, this is the hair that frames your forehead. It can be worn long, short, or anything in between.

DISCONNECT

In relation to undercuts, this refers to the difference in length between the hair on top of your head to that on the sides. This difference needs to be at least an inch (2.5 cm) so that there is a clear visual distinction between the sides and top. See also *Undercut*.

DUTCH BRAID

The same as a French braid (plait), but in reverse. Rather than the strands passing over into the center of the braid to produce an inverted braid, the strands pass under and up to produce a braid that sits close to the head but stands up from it.

FADE

A style that is shorter at the back and sides and longer on top, with the hair length tapering gradually from one length to the other. See also *Undercut*.

FRENCH BRAID

A variation on the standard three-strand braid (plait) that "hugs" the scalp. Three small strands of hair start off the braid at the top, and these strands then incorporate hair from either side of the head as the braid progresses, producing an inverted braid. See also *Dutch braid*.

HAIR CUTICLE

The outermost protective layer of a strand of hair, consisting of a series of overlapping scales. Blow-drying down the length of the hair shaft will encourage these scales to lie flat, thereby giving a smooth, shiny appearance. Hair colors and other chemical treatments work by penetrating this outer layer, which is why they can sometimes be damaging to the hair.

HAIR SHAFT

The portion of a strand of hair that is visible above the skin. A strand of hair grows out of a follicle that sits below the skin. See also hair cuticle.

LINING A BEARD

Essentially, creating a clean, neat outline for your beard to determine its shape. A well-defined beard needs to be lined along the cheeks, the jaw, and under the chin—and right up to the sideburns, if that's the style you're going for.

OCCIPITAL BONE

The bone that sits at the back of your head, just above your neck—the area where the base of a low ponytail sits.

PIECING

Adding texture by separating out small sections of hair and defining them individually with product and/or your fingers.

POMPADOUR

A style where the hair is swept up and back. The sides are slicked straight back, while the top of the hair sits high above the forehead. This style was particularly popular during the 1950s and '60s, so is perfect for creating a retro look.

QUIFF

A term that sometimes gets used interchangeably with "pompadour." Both styles sit high on the head at the front, but a pompadour is always slicked back, whereas a quiff can have a lot more texture and volume.

THREE-STRAND BRAID

Also known as a plait, this technique involves dividing the hair into three equal sections and then alternately passing the strands on either side over and into the center of the braid. This method is also the basis for more complex variations, such as a *French braid* and a *Dutch braid*.

UNDERCUT

A style that is longer on top, and shorter at the sides and back, with a distinct difference in length between these two areas, although the lengths of both can vary. See also *Fade*.

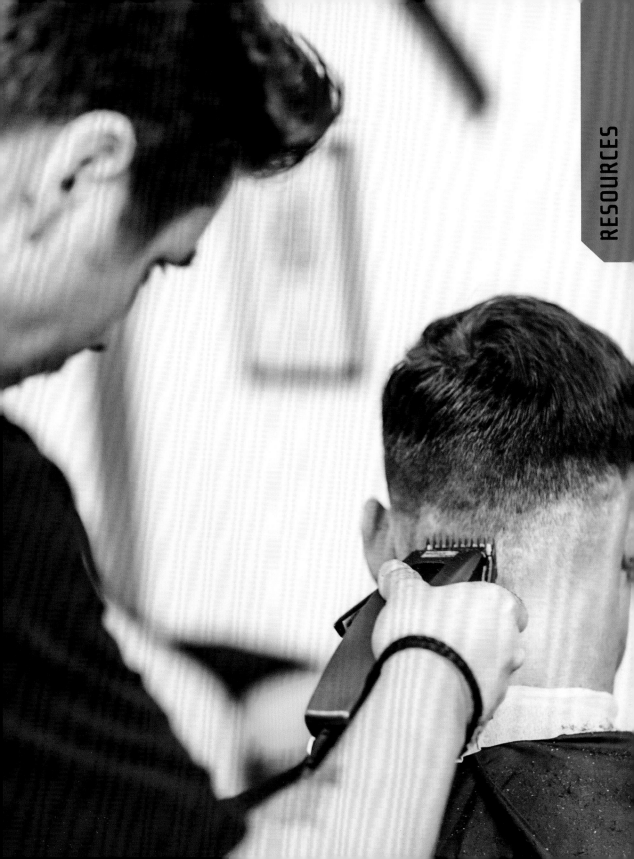

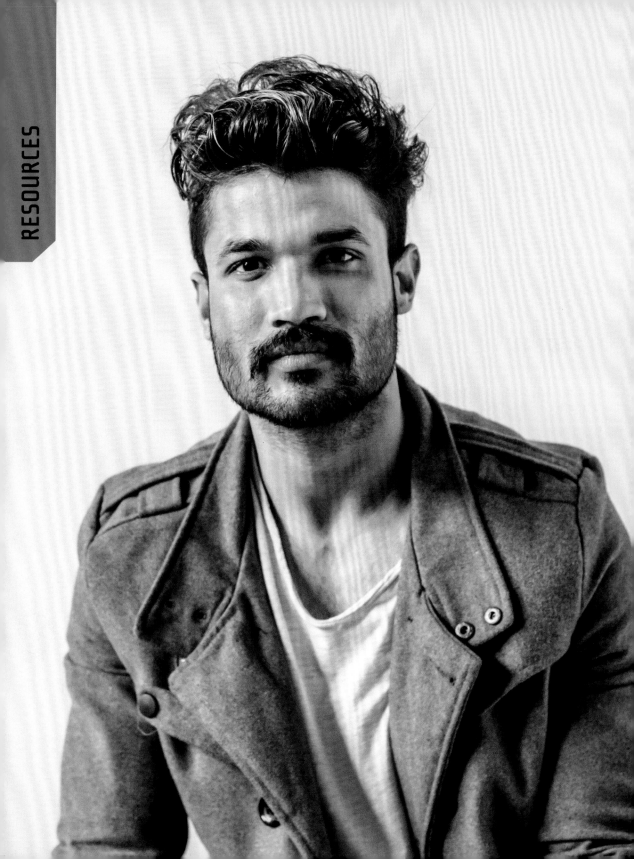

SUPPLIERS

Once you enter the world of products and tools, you'll realize just how much is out there. You will discover that there are literally hundreds of different products for your hair and beard—with many different names. What I have referred to as fiber paste, for example, might be sold as "putty" or "clay," and one pomade is not necessarily the same as the next. To add to the confusion, the same thing may also be given different names by different brands.

Tools are also a world unto themselves, with all sorts of brands offering their own versions of the basics. But don't worry—once you start to explore the options you will soon narrow it down to what works for you. You may make mistakes, but then that's how you learn.

The following are just some of the brands that I used to create the styles in this book, which you may want to check out. But don't feel restricted to what I use—with so many options available, at so many different price points, it's worth shopping around.

If in doubt, always ask your barber or stylist for recommendations. They will be able to give you personalized advice, and will usually stock a number of products that you can try before you buy.

BABYLISS

This company produces a wide selection of good-quality styling tools, from beard trimmers and flat irons to hair dryers. You'll also find mini-beard trimmers, like the one I've used to create a few of the 'taches and beards in this book, and mini flat irons, for working on small sections of hair at a time.

DENMAN

Denman produce a number of brushes at reasonable prices, from classic styling brushes through to vent brushes and wide paddle brushes. They also supply combs and Afro picks.

MASON PEARSON

If you want to invest in a top-of-the-range brush, then I would recommend a nylon/boar-bristle combination brush from Mason Pearson. They are a lot more expensive than an average drugstore brush, but will last you a lifetime if you take proper care of them. The brush features a mix of boar bristles (slightly shorter) and nylon bristles (slightly longer), and is suitable for medium to thick hair.

PRO-TIP

Pro-Tip offer a number of professional-quality combs, from small-tooth up to wide-tooth, and a few in between. Look out for combs that are small-toothed at one end and wide-toothed at the other if you don't want to purchase too many tools. A comb with a long end as a handle can also be handy for creating parts in your hair.

TIGI

TIGI supply stores and salons with a vast selection of professional-grade haircare and styling products. I particularly like their salt spray, which I used for a number of the styles in this book.

LYNX

If you are looking for reliable, no-nonsense styling products, LYNX are a good place to start, especially if you are wanting to experiment with different textured finishes and levels of hold. Drugstore products provide an affordable way to explore your options before committing to salon-quality alternatives.

USEFUL RESOURCES

My hope is that what I've provided in the pages of this book is enough for you to be able to create any of the styles demonstrated here, and many more besides, using your newfound skills.

However, I also want to encourage you to start looking around for inspiration, instruction, and clarification for yourself. Guys are becoming more and more interested in hair styling and personal grooming, and as a result there is a massive amount of information now available for free online, whether it's hair care, tips on facial-hair grooming, or how-to tutorials for all sorts of styles. A quick online search will almost always give you the answers that you're looking for.

THELONDONBARBER.COM

This is my own website, which is focused at the moment on education, so if you're in the UK and interested in taking your skills further, check it out. Even if you're not, you'll find plenty of inspiration on there just by scrolling through some of the projects I've worked on. My ultimate aim is for this to become a men's lifestyle brand, and several hair products are in the pipeline, so watch this space!

INSTAGRAM

Looking at pictures of what your celeb heroes are doing with their hair will keep you up to date with the latest trends. And a few of the models used in this book have massive Instagram followings, so if you like their style, it might be worth keeping an eye on what they're doing.

As I've stressed before, though, while it's worth taking inspiration from them, it's important to stay true to yourself and choose those styles that really express who you are. Don't waste time wishing that you had someone else's hair—if you have confidence and embrace your own strengths, then people will start copying YOU!

YOUTUBE

It sounds obvious, but you'll be amazed at what you can find on YouTube. If I'm curious about a particular technique, I will always check out what's online—there's bound to be someone somewhere who's done a tutorial on it. You need to use a bit of common sense, though. Not everyone is an expert, and there is lots of bad in with the good. You just need to take note of the people who are producing good results. Check out Jim Chapman, for example. He offers accessible and reliable tips and tutorials relating to both fashion and hair. And there are dozens of interesting bloggers out there, covering hair techniques, product reviews, style advice, and more.

GQ

I don't read a lot of magazines, but this is a great one for style and fashion inspiration. It's important to think of hair in context—how it works with clothing and fits in with the culture.

MODERN BARBER

This is a magazine for industry professionals, but it's worth looking at even if you aren't a barber yourself. You can browse through and pick up on the latest techniques, and you will also be able to read about the barbers in your area.

SALONS

Any hairdressing salon will always have a pile of hair and fashion magazines available for their customers, so if you decide to visit a stylist, go with some extra time beforehand so that you can rifle through the pages for ideas.

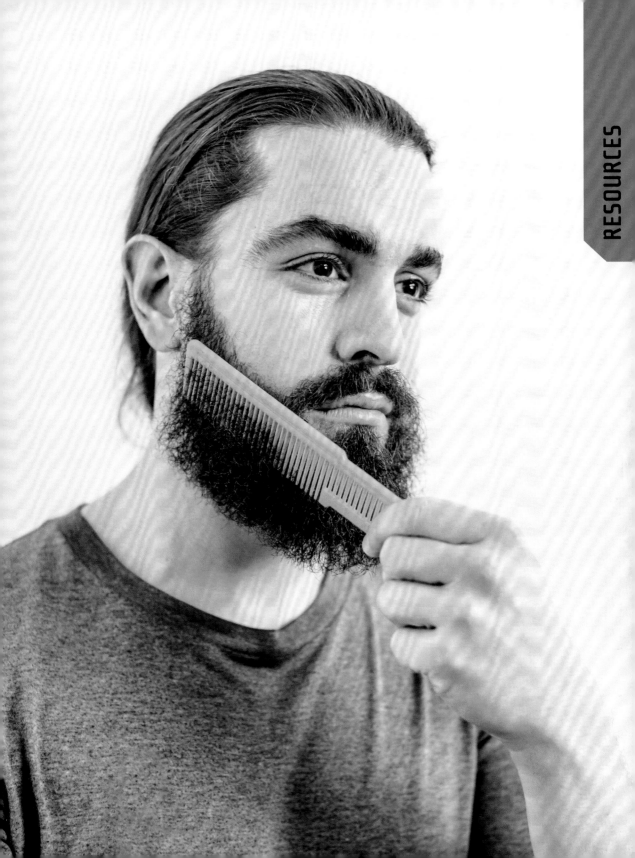

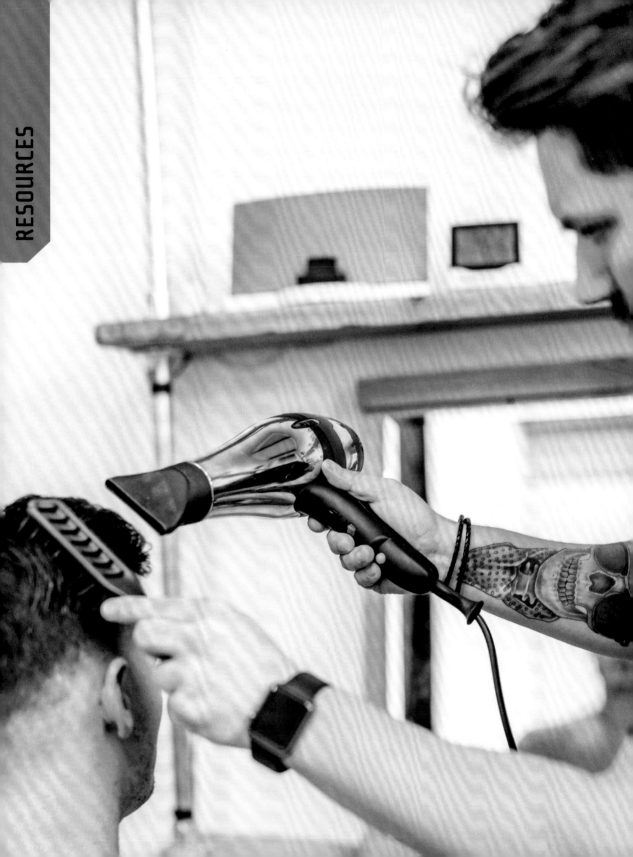

CONTRIBUTORS & CREDITS

HAIR STYLIST
Kieron Webb

LOCATION PHOTOGRAPHY
Neal Grundy
Emma Gutteridge

MAKEUP
Jen Morrell
Hannah Davies

MODELS
Frankie Andrews
(pages 64–65, 74–75)

Waz Ashayer
(pages 44–45, 72–73)

Adam Bond
(pages 84–85, 98–99, 114–115,
122–123, 128–129)

Philip Bottenberg
(pages 92–93, 126–127, 140–141)

Roy Brackpool
(pages 82–83, 130–131)

Tommy Brady
(pages 58–59, 66–67, 134–135)

Krasen Dimitrov
(pages 42–43)

Lloydd Harwijk
(pages 88–89, 96–97, 132–133)

Sam Hume
(pages 36–37, 50–51, 78–79)

Scott Kean
(pages 90–91, 94–95, 100–101,
108–109)

Steve Laurence
(pages 70–71)

Myles Leask
(pages 38–39, 48–49, 144–147)

Joshua Mascolo
(pages 104–105, 118–119)

Alvaro Augusto Ramos Neto
(pages 54–55, 136–137, 142–143)

Axel Nu
(pages 86–87, 102–103, 112–113)

Nathan Pearce
(pages 40–41)

Sean Prakash
(pages 68–69)

Konrad Szwarczynski
(pages 76–77)

Glain Varghese
(pages 46–47, 62–63, 150–151,
158–159, 162–163)

Kieron Webb
(pages 154–155)

Joseph Knowles
(pages 106–107)

OTHER IMAGES
Getty Images
12 (all), 34 (top right and bottom
left), 80 (top right and bottom left),
116 (top left and bottom right), 148
(top left and top right), 153, 161,
164 (top left)

Shutterstock
19, 53, 57, 124, 164 (bottom right)

Stocksy
32, 34 (top left and bottom left), 61,
111, 116 (top right), 120, 138, 148
(bottom left and bottom right), 157,
164 (top right and bottom left)

Alamy
80 (top left and bottom right), 116

Joseph Knowles
107

INDEX

ACKNOWLEDGMENTS

ACKNOWLEDGMENTS

This book has been one of the hardest and most testing projects I have ever worked on, but it has also been one of the highlights of my career journey so far. I would like to start by saying a massive thank you to my amazing girlfriend Alice, for her love, support, patience, and positive energy throughout the entire process. Behind every project is a great team of people who make the whole thing happen, so I would also like to thank Jen and Hannah for all their hard work, grooming the lads; Emma and Neil for capturing the cuts and styles so brilliantly; and Angela for editing and making sure that this Cockney lad sounded articulate! Thank you, finally, to the team at RotoVision for giving me this opportunity—it has truly been a fantastic experience.

BIOGRAPHY

Kieron Webb is The London Barber. He created The London Barber as a hairstyling education brand, designed to train aspiring barbers and hairdressers based on the expertise and technical skills that he has built up over more than a decade in the industry. The London Barber is also a way for Kieron to educate men of all ages when it comes to the tricks of the trade—showing them how to use salon techniques to achieve their desired styles.

Kieron has become a highly sought-after stylist, working regularly with celebrity clients such as Zayn Malik; YouTube star Joe Sugg; leading fashion designer, and CEO of Ralph&Russo, Michael Russo; and artist manager/TV producer Simon Fuller, to name a few. Kieron also works regularly with the renowned photographer Joseph Sinclair, capturing famous faces for magazine editorials.

Since the launch of The London Barber, Kieron has signed for LYNX as Global Creative Director, a role that has seen him create styles for the brand's global advertising campaigns. This role also led to Kieron heading the hair team for top young fashion designers Agi&Sam's SS/17 and AW/17 runway shows at London Collections Men.